THE COMPLETE WOMEN'S GUIDE TO PEPTIDES

CUTTING-EDGE BIOHACKING PEPTIDE
THERAPY TO RESTORE ENERGY, BALANCE
HORMONES, BURN FAT, ENHANCE NATURAL
BEAUTY, AND BOOST LONGEVITY

SAGE O'REILLEY

THE EMERALD
SOCIETY

LEAVE A REVIEW

Don't forget to share the love and **leave your
<u>Amazon review</u>** for:

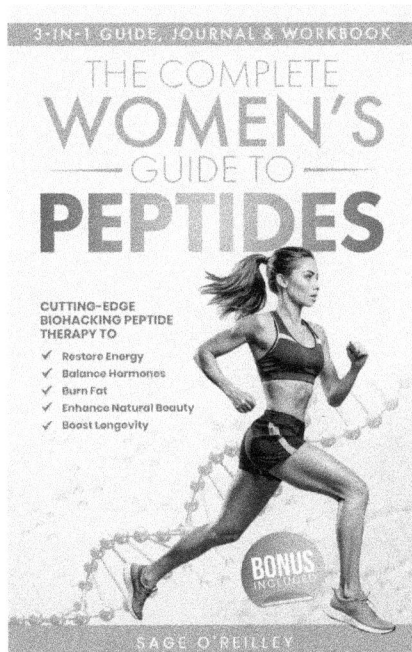

CONTENTS

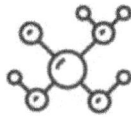

PEPTIDE HACKS

Biohacking with peptides is a modern, science-backed approach to supporting our body's natural functions.

Using tiny chains of amino acids (aka peptides), we can personalize wellness for hormone balance, weight management, improved metabolic function, skin repair, and mental clarity.

For us women, it is a powerful and precise way to reclaim control of our health and aging on a cellular level.

Y.D. GARDENS

PREFACE

Dear fearless biohacker,

Before you dive into the life-changing world of peptides, I need to give you a quick heads-up.

This book is all about sharing knowledge, research, and the latest on biohacking with peptides. Think of it as your personal toolkit for understanding how these little protein powerhouses work.

Peptides are seriously powerful, and their effects on your body deserve attention. That's why it's essential to consult with a qualified medical professional before you start experimenting with any peptide protocol. I'm talking about those amazing docs or health experts who can guide you, track your progress, and ensure everything you're doing is in sync with your body's unique needs.

While I'm here to provide the knowledge, you're the one who gets to make the empowered, well-informed decisions. And, once you do, you'll be on your way to feeling like the healthiest, most energized version of yourself.

Bottom line: This book is packed with all the peptide goodness you could ever want, but when it comes to putting those insights into action, always check in with a pro. And don't worry: Just by reading through, you're already ahead of the game! You'll be armed with an abundance of knowledge to make informed choices and understand how peptides can play a role in your wellness journey.

So, flip that page, keep reading, and let's dive into the fascinating world of peptides.

— *Sage*

INTRODUCTION

IT'S 2 A.M., AND THE BLUE LIGHT OF YOUR PHONE IS THE ONLY thing lighting up the dark. Your mind is racing. You scroll through endless forums, looking for that one magic answer. You've tried every clean-eating plan, every supplement, every "miracle" fix recommended by that one friend on social media who seems to have a solution for everything. Still, you wake up tired, feel bloated, and can't quite remember the last time you felt like your old self.

Maybe you know this woman. Maybe she's you. You take care of everyone else (your family, your job, your friends), but when's the last time you took care of you? You're running on fumes, wishing for more energy, better sleep, a body that *actually* feels like it's working with you instead of against you.

You're done with the confusion.

You just want answers.

I've met hundreds of women in this exact spot. I am, amongst other things, a naturopath who's a little obsessed with helping women get their spark back. But here's where my Peptide journey started: A client in my early days. A sleep-deprived mom who stumbled into my office looking like she'd been living off caffeine and willpower for far too long. Her hair was thinning, her energy was nonexistent, and she had been told by doctors that her labs were "normal." But honestly, nothing felt normal for her.

Together, we ventured deeper. We took a hard look at how her body, mind, and lifestyle were connected. With a few strategic changes (including some targeted peptides) we were able to turn things around. She started sleeping through the night, thinking clearly, and waking up with energy. And I watched that transformation unfold and thought, *I need to do this more. I need to help more women feel this way.*

Over the past decades, I've worked with women from all walks of life: new moms, busy professionals, athletes, and grandmas. Time passes, but one thing never changes: The health and wellness world is overloaded with advice. But a lot of it is geared toward men, or worse, built on questionable science. When it comes to biohacking, the gap is even wider. There are a ton of guides and protocols, but most ignore the unique biology, hormones, and goals of women. They rarely speak to our needs or our rhythms.

This book? It's here to change that.

You deserve a toolbox built just for you, and that's why I wrote *A Woman's Guide to Biohacking with Peptides.* This is a practical resource designed to help you use peptides safely and effectively. Every protocol, every tip, every explanation is aimed at helping you feel better, without getting tangled up in jargon or lost in a sea of confusing options.

Peptides are much more than just some buzzword. They're tiny chains of amino acids that act as messengers in your body. Over the past few years, research has shown how these natural compounds can help with energy, hormone balance, fat loss, skin health, and even aging. But here's the kicker: peptides are a true game-changer for women who feel overlooked by mainstream solutions. Whether you want to wake up feeling more rested, shed that stubborn weight, age beautifully from the inside out, or simply feel like yourself again, peptides can help you get there.

Now, I know it's tough to sort fact from fiction. The internet is full of big promises, sketchy advice, and people throwing around words like "revolutionary" and "miracle" without any real science behind them. Some sources make peptides sound risky, or like you have to be some kind of PhD wizard to use them. But here's my promise to you: *This book cuts through the noise.* I break it all down in ways that are easy to understand and apply. I've included real-life stories, checklists, safety tips, and step-by-step guides you can start using right away.

So, what's inside? First, we're going to make the science simple. I'll explain what peptides are, how they work, and why they're worth your attention. Then, we'll cover how to safely source them and avoid common mistakes. You'll get clear protocols for things like restoring energy, balancing hormones, burning fat, and even enhancing your beauty (hello, glowing skin!). Each chapter builds on the last, so you'll have a plan tailored to your unique needs and goals. As a bonus, each section will include a point-by-point summary of the key takeaways, for easier understanding and future reference. Plus, I'll show you how to track your progress and adjust as life changes (because life *always* changes, right?).

By the end of this book, I want you to feel empowered, confident, and ready to take control of your health, not just for now, but for years to come. This is not just another book; it's a tool to help you build your best self.

I've written this with love, years of listening to women just like you, and a whole lot of passion for helping others feel strong, clear-headed, and alive. If you've ever felt brushed aside by mainstream advice, or if you're just ready to try something new and science-backed, I invite you to join me in this journey. We're going to explore the cutting edge of peptide therapy in a way that's approachable, safe, and most importantly, inspiring.

Your story doesn't end with fatigue or frustration; it ends with you thriving.

ONE
DEMYSTIFYING PEPTIDES FOR THE MODERN WOMAN

You know that feeling when you stare at your reflection after a rough night, tracing the lines around your eyes and wondering, "There must be a better way to feel like myself again"? I remember talking with a friend over coffee, her voice hushed as she confessed she'd spent hours researching anti-aging creams and energy supplements, only to end up more confused than ever. She wanted to feel energized, focused, and confident in her own skin, but kept bumping into the same tired advice. Maybe you've been there too, caught between wellness trends and medical jargon, feeling like the real answers are hidden just out of reach. That's where I started too, both as a woman and as a practitioner. So, I propose we cut through the noise and discover the real story on peptides.

Peptides 101: What Every Woman Needs to Know

Let's get right to the heart of it: Peptides are not some new-age invention or mysterious "biohacker" tool. At their core, peptides are short chains of amino acids; think of them as the building blocks that make up proteins. But what is so special about them is how they act as messengers in your body. If you picture your body as a busy office, peptides are the quick text messages sent between coworkers to make things happen fast. When you cut your finger, for example, certain peptides signal your cells to start the repair process. They don't waste time with long meetings; they send a direct order: "Fix this now." In fact, collagen peptides, which you may have seen in beauty powders or creams, are probably already part of your daily routine. Those collagen peptides help support firmer skin and stronger hair by telling your body to boost its own natural collagen production.

Peptides play an astonishing range of roles in your health. They're involved in nearly everything you care about: how quickly you heal after a tough workout, how rested you feel in the morning, whether your cravings spiral out of control before your period, and how radiant your skin looks after a few nights of good sleep. Let's break it down with real-life examples. When you scrape your knee or heal from surgery, peptides spring into action by instructing your body to patch up the damage. If you're tossing and turning all night or waking up hungry at 2 a.m., it's often because peptides are sending signals that affect your sleep hormones or appetite cues. Even that surge of energy after a refreshing walk? Peptides help regulate the hormones responsible for alertness and mood.

Biohacking with peptides might sound intimidating at first, but here's the truth: You're probably already biohacking every time you tweak your skincare, adjust your supplements, or play with nutrition to see what helps you feel better. Using peptides is just another way of giving your body the right messages at the right time, a more targeted method for supporting what you already do. You don't need to be an athlete or a scientist; you simply need curiosity and a willingness to listen to your own body. I've coached women who started off as skeptics, worried they might get lost in scientific lingo or do something "wrong." One client confessed she was worried about "messing up her hormones" but became one of my most confident peptide users after we walked through protocols together.

I understand if all of this feels new or even a bit overwhelming. Peptides aren't just for scientists in lab coats or gym buffs chasing muscle gains. You belong here in this conversation just as much as anyone else. Women have unique rhythms: our hormones shift throughout our cycles and our lives, which means our needs are different from men's. That's why it's so important for us to claim this space and learn how peptides can be used safely and wisely. You can absolutely understand this field, and you can absolutely use these tools in a way that fits your life.

Key Takeaways...

Peptides Are the Body's Instant Messaging System:
Peptides are short chains of amino acids that act as messengers in your body, giving direct orders for healing, energy, and skin health.

Peptides Help Heal, Feel Energized, and Glow:
From boosting collagen for firmer skin to regulating sleep hormones and keeping cravings in check, peptides support everything from workout recovery to that radiant morning glow.

Biohacking with Peptides is for Every Woman:
You don't need to be a scientist or a fitness fanatic to benefit from peptides. It's simply a smarter way to support your wellness routine.

Peptides Aren't As Complicated As They Seem: Peptides

are easy to use, and with a little curiosity, you'll be a pro in no time. Don't let the science intimidate you—you're in control!

Peptide Insights

Pause for a moment and ask yourself:

Where do I feel stuck with my energy or wellness right now?

What would it mean for me to have clear steps not just for "getting by," but for actually feeling like myself again?

_____

_____

_____

_____

_____

_____

_____

_____

_____

_____

_____

_____

Peptide therapy has been used for decades. Insulin is one of the earliest examples, first used in the 1920s for diabetes. Since then, scientists have developed dozens of other peptides for everything from healing injuries to improving memory. The key is that peptides are not a fad; they're a powerful part of how our bodies communicate and repair themselves every single day. You have every right to explore this field with confidence and curiosity.

The Body's Natural Peptides

Your body naturally produces a variety of peptides that quietly regulate your daily wellbeing. Take oxytocin, commonly known as the "love hormone." The warm, safe feeling you get when holding your child, hugging a friend, or bonding with a pet? That's oxytocin at work, calming your nervous system, reducing stress, boosting healing, and strengthening your emotional connections and resilience.

Mood swings and bursts of happiness also have a biological basis. Endorphins, another peptide group, function as mood elevators. They're released during activities like exercise, eating chocolate, or laughing, reducing pain and lifting your spirits—explaining that euphoric high after a workout. Balanced endorphin levels help you handle stress, recover from life's setbacks, and better manage the ups and downs of hormonal changes.

Then there's insulin, perhaps better known, but easily overlooked as a peptide. It moves sugar from the blood into your cells for energy, especially after a carb-heavy meal or a sweet treat. When insulin functions well, energy remains steady and the mind is clear. But stress, poor sleep, or hormonal shifts can disrupt insulin's effect, causing energy dips and cravings. Keeping peptides balanced is essential, as they help guide your mood, focus, and metabolism.

Peptide production changes throughout life. During puberty,

peptides coordinate the surge of hormones and bodily changes; in pregnancy, oxytocin and other peptides spike to foster bonding and prepare for childbirth. Menstruation triggers peptide-driven signals affecting mood, appetite, and energy. The greatest shift occurs around menopause, when estrogen and collagen peptide levels drop, leading to thinner skin, slower healing, and dips in energy. These are not just signs of aging but reflect shifts in peptide production that impact everything from recovery and weight management to mental clarity.

Weight shifts, premenstrual moods, or skin changes after forty are all linked to natural peptide fluctuations. When peptide levels decline due to menopause, chronic stress, or aging, women experience more than just hot flashes or wrinkles. Bruising easily, slow energy recovery after illness, or delayed wound healing? Peptide decline often plays a role. Even PMS mood swings are connected to the interplay of peptides with hormones like serotonin and progesterone.

The key insight: peptide therapy doesn't try to override your body, instead offering gentle encouragement to restore natural balance. Think of it as supporting internal signals that may have faded with age or stress, not hacking your biology. You're helping your system do what it's designed for, restoring your vitality, not forcing artificial change.

Peptide optimization is ideal for women because it works with your constantly shifting internal chemistry throughout life's cycles and stages. Rather than over-relying on outside hormones or endless supplements, peptide therapy supports your natural processes, restoring balance where things have slowed. Women's needs evolve, so understanding and partnering with your chemistry lets you address fatigue, slow recovery, stubborn weight gain, or mood lows in a way that suits your unique life phase.

When introducing women to peptide therapy, I emphasize it's not about force or radical change, but a subtle nudge. You aren't rewriting your body's instructions; you're simply reactivating clear signals that may have diminished with time. This makes peptide therapy appealing to women who want to remain active and energized, honoring their natural rhythms as they age.

Life Stages & Peptide Shifts

The following chart illustrates the fluctuations of oxytocin, endorphins, insulin, and collagen peptides across different life stages. Notice how peptide levels change during puberty, pregnancy, menstruation, menopause, and aging. This represents how fluctuations in these peptides may correlate with symptoms like mood swings, slower healing, and skin changes at each stage.

Ultimately, peptide therapy is about partnering with your own biology and supporting the intrinsic wisdom of your cells to offer a gentle boost when your system needs it most.

How Peptides Differ from Supplements, Hormones, and Pharmaceuticals

Supplements work like fuel, providing the vitamins and minerals your body needs to function smoothly. Hormones act as high-level managers, controlling large systems and causing sweeping changes. Peptides, on the other hand, are like concise, targeted text messages passed between departments. Their job is to deliver specific instructions—such as "start repairing tissue here" or "boost skin renewal"—and then quickly vanish.

Here is a table to show, for example, the differences between Vitamin C, Estrogen Therapy, and BPC-157 Peptide.

Vitamin C vs Estrogen Therapy vs BPC-157 Peptide

Material	Vitamin C	Estrogen Therapy	BPC-157 Peptide
Type	Vitamin	Hormone	Peptide
Benefits	Antioxidant	Menopausal symptom relief	Promotes healing
Routes	Oral, topical	Oral, transdermal	Injection

Supplements top up our resources but rarely create big changes on their own. Hormones can bring substantial benefits but may also cause broad side effects. Estrogen therapy, for example, can help with hot flashes yet also alters mood, breast tissue, and more. Peptides work differently. They slip in, deliver their exact instructions to a single process, and then break down. This precise action means peptides cause fewer unintended effects and don't disturb other systems in your body.

This targeted approach is a key strength of peptides. Take BPC-157: if you overextend your knee during exercise, this peptide can prompt your body to speed up repair exactly where it's needed. Compare that to ibuprofen, which dulls inflammation throughout the body, sometimes slowing healing and irritating your stomach too. BPC-157 focuses its action solely where it's needed, causing fewer side effects and less overall disruption—like changing just one radio channel instead of lowering the volume on the whole stereo.

When used correctly, peptides usually avoid the broad, systemic changes of hormones. Adjusting your estrogen or thyroid levels can alter mood, metabolism, and reproductive health, sometimes all at once. Peptides work in smaller, focused bursts, mimicking the body's natural signals. Their familiar structure allows for smooth integration when they're used as intended and sourced from quality providers.

Many women I work with wonder if peptides are just another supplement or perhaps something unnatural. In reality, they're already familiar—collagen peptides in beauty products support your skin by nudging your body to make more collagen where you need it. Hormone therapies, by contrast, impact every cell in your body that's sensitive to those hormones and can bring widespread effects. For example, while both peptides and hormones can help with skin aging, peptides do so gently and locally, not by shifting your body's entire hormonal landscape.

Here's a scenario: maybe you've tried collagen peptides in your morning smoothie and noticed smoother skin. If, however, you're healing slowly after surgery or injury, a targeted peptide like BPC-157 might speed up recovery at the site of injury without causing problems elsewhere, unlike broad supplements or systemic medication.

Keep in mind that peptides aren't magic bullets or substitutes for good basics like nutrition and medical care. Consider them precision tools for addressing particular health concerns without broad-stroke, whole-body solutions.

Here's a simplified approach:

- Are you eating well, moving, and sleeping enough, but still facing a specific health issue?
    - If your concern is broad (like general fatigue), review your nutrition and lifestyle first.
    - If it's specific (like slow injury recovery or deep wrinkles), a targeted peptide may help.
- Considering hormones? Always discuss with your doctor, weighing the pros and cons.

      ○ If you seek gentler, more focused action, peptides may be the middle ground.

Ultimately, peptides are suited for a layered health approach that starts with basics like nutritious food, exercise, sleep, and stress management. If those aren't enough, peptides offer a next step: precise, advanced signals to tackle stubborn, localized problems. They're not miracle cures or household supplements, but another tool to help you shape your health intentionally and effectively.

The Science Behind Peptide Biohacking

Every woman I know wants to feel like she's making smart choices for her body, not just guessing and hoping for the best. Science can feel like a wall you have to climb just to get the answers you need, especially when it comes to something as new-sounding as peptide therapy. I want you to feel at ease, so let's break it down together. Picture a peptide as a key and your body's many tiny cell receptors as locks. Each lock only opens for a certain key. When you introduce a peptide, it fits into its matching lock, turning it just so, and triggers a specific action—maybe it signals your cells to start repairing muscle after a tough workout or tells skin cells to boost their own collagen production. This "lock and key" fit is why peptides are so targeted. They don't wander around causing mayhem; they look for their match and then quietly do their job.

But not every key finds its lock with the same ease, which is where "bioavailability" comes in. When taking a vitamin pill, only some of what you swallow actually gets absorbed and reaches where it's needed. Bioavailability is simply the measure of how much of a peptide you use actually makes it to those cell locks, ready to turn them on. While some peptides are easily absorbed through the skin or gut, others need to be injected because stomach acids would break them down before they ever reach their target.

You might wonder if all this is just theory or if real research backs up these claims. The answer is that peptides are being studied in labs and clinics all over the world, with results that are both promising and relevant for women. BPC-157, for example, has been shown to speed up recovery from muscle injuries by directing repair signals exactly where they're needed. Another peptide, CJC-1295, stimulates your own growth hormone release, which can mean better muscle tone, faster metabolism, and deeper sleep, all without the risks of taking straight-up hormones. These miracle molecules are tested in real settings and show measurable shifts in how women feel and function.

Safety and dosing are where many women start to worry, and rightly so. You'll want protocols that feel approachable, not mysterious or dangerous. The principle here is simple: **start low, go slow**. More is not always better with peptides. Taking a huge dose won't double your results, it may just overwhelm your system or waste expensive product. Small, measured steps give your body time to respond and let you notice changes without risk. Protocols often begin with the lowest recommended dose for a short period, followed by gentle increases only if needed and tolerated. If you're new to peptides, this approach will let you observe subtle shifts (better energy, improved sleep quality, or easier recovery) while staying safe.

Designing protocols isn't about copying what worked for someone else on Instagram; every woman's biology is unique. Age, weight, hormonal status, stress levels—all these matter. For example, if you're peri-menopausal and struggling with sleep disruption and stubborn belly fat, your peptide needs may look different from someone training for a marathon or healing after surgery. Protocol selection starts with your goals (energy restoration, fat loss, cognitive clarity) and then tailors dosing and timing based on what your body tells you.

Science is always moving forward, so it's important to separate what we know from what's still being explored. Some peptides, like insulin or collagen fragments, have decades of proven safety and efficacy behind them. Others (think BPC-157 for tissue repair or CJC-1295 for metabolic health) have solid early evidence from animal studies and small human trials, but aren't yet household names among doctors. There are also a few peptides marketed online that are still experimental, and while their effects may be exciting, they are not fully understood or regulated yet.

In a Nutshell...

Peptides are targeted "keys" that fit into your body's "locks" (cell receptors) to trigger specific actions like muscle repair or collagen production.

Bioavailability is how much of the peptide actually reaches its target. Some need injections, others can be absorbed through your skin or gut.

Real research backs up peptides: They're being studied and tested, with proven results.

Safety first: Start slow, go low. Don't rush to higher doses. Allow your body to adjust safely and effectively.

. . .

Personalized protocols are key: Your peptide plan should be as unique as you are. Consider your age, goals, and lifestyle to choose the right approach.

Not all peptides are created equal: Some have decades of proven benefits, while others are still being researched. Keep an eye on what's been studied and what's still in the early stages.

What's Proven, What's Promising, What's Not Ready Yet

Peptide	Evidence Level	Application
Insulin	Proven	Blood sugar control
Collagen peptides	Promising	Skin health
BPC-157	Promising	Injury recovery
CJC-1295	Promising	Growth hormone support
Melanotan II	Not Ready Yet	Tanning

Reliable research matters most when your health is on the line. Trust what's been shown safe in repeat studies and watch for updates on newer therapies that could soon become part of everyday care for women like you. There's power in understanding both the potential and the limits, because when you know what each peptide can do (and what it can't), you're equipped to make informed decisions without fear or confusion.

Why do Women Biohack?

Frankly, most of us step into biohacking out of necessity. Fatigue seeps into the bones, mornings blur into each other, and despite your best efforts (clean eating, supplements, exercise), the old spark remains elusive. What really drives this search isn't some shallow desire for perfection, it's a deep need to feel like yourself again. Energy is precious when you're juggling work deadlines, family schedules, and your own emotional tides. You might notice the shift in your thirties or forties, when sleep becomes lighter, stubborn pounds creep in, or focus slips away just when you need it most.

Many women I meet say the same thing: **"I just want my mind sharp and my body steady. I want to feel present**." The traditional advice—one-size-fits-all diets, generic supplements, vague encouragement to "manage stress"—often falls flat. We crave solutions that genuinely fit our lives, our cycles, and our changing bodies.

We also know that the pain points run much deeper than physical symptoms. Hormonal complexity can turn each month into a guessing game. Maybe you've hit a plateau after months of effort, only to be told to try harder or "wait it out." In male-dominated biohacking spaces, women's experiences get sidelined or dismissed altogether. There's a frustration that comes from reading protocols built for men and realizing they don't translate. You're left piecing together fragments of advice, hoping something will stick. The reality is that women's bodies respond differently—to stress, to exercise, to aging—and the old playbook doesn't honor that. Peptide biohacking offers an answer, allowing for protocols that support hormonal balance, skin renewal, cognitive clarity, and steady energy through every life phase.

Stories from real women bring these points to life far better than any abstract promise. I remember working with a nurse in her early forties who loved her job but felt drained by her shifts. She'd tried every "energy booster" on the market but still woke up exhausted. When we introduced a peptide protocol designed for metabolic support and recovery, she noticed a real shift within weeks. Her colleagues commented on her new glow; she had energy left for her family after twelve-hour days.

Another client, a mother of two, had given up running after a stubborn ankle injury that refused to heal despite months of therapy. She felt stuck, like her body was betraying her love for movement. With a targeted peptide regimen focused on tissue repair, her healing accelerated. Six months later, she texted me a sweaty selfie from the finish line of her first 5K since the injury.

But before-and-after moments aren't just about numbers on a scale or clocking faster miles. They're about reclaiming lost confidence, feeling in sync with your own body again, and knowing you have tools that actually adapt to your needs. Women who once described themselves as "foggy" or "invisible" began to speak up at work meetings or sign up for new adventures because their minds felt clear and their bodies resilient. Plateaus faded when protocols shifted with hormonal cycles instead of fighting against them. Night sweats eased, skin brightened, and so did relationships, because energy returned not just physically but emotionally.

What stands out most is the sense of autonomy. With peptides, you set the pace. This process also has the potential to forge powerful connections with other women, whether in private Facebook groups, local meetups, or even text threads with friends trying new protocols together. One woman told me, "I never thought I'd feel so seen or supported just by sharing my experience with peptides." The community aspect dissolves isolation and builds confidence. Hard-won wisdom gets passed around: what worked during perimenopause, how to adjust peptides before travel, which changes were subtle but meaningful.

.   .   .

Quotes from these women often echo in my mind:

"I feel like I finally have a say in how I age."

"Peptides made me realize I'm not broken; my body just needed something different."

"Sharing my results gave me courage to try things I'd written off for years."

These are the stories of women reclaiming their lives on their own terms. For many, peptide protocols become an act of self-mastery and self-respect. It's a refusal to settle for fatigue or frustration as the new normal. It's about building a toolkit that evolves with you, honors your complexity, and connects you to others on the same path toward vitality and renewal.

Busting Myths and Separating Hype from Reality

There's a moment that hits many women right before they press "buy" on a peptide product or even mention peptide therapy at their next checkup, a tangle of doubts and "what ifs." I hear it all the time. Isn't this stuff illegal? Aren't peptides just for hardcore gym rats? Do I need a biochemistry degree to use them safely? The fear of being duped by slick marketing or wasting money on snake oil is real. If you've ever found yourself eyeing a bottle and wondering if you're being sold a dream, you're not alone. This world is full of big promises and half-truths, and nobody wants to feel foolish or, worse, unsafe.

Let's clear the slate with honesty. First, the myth that "peptides are illegal" comes up everywhere. In reality, legality depends on where you live and how peptides are marketed or used. Many peptides are available through licensed healthcare providers for medical purposes. Others can be legally purchased as research chemicals in some countries, while a few are tightly regulated. It's true you should never trust a source that doesn't provide clear information about purity, testing, and legal status. But using peptides under professional supervision is not breaking the law, and you aren't doing anything shady by wanting to explore these therapies for your own wellbeing.

The second big myth is that you need to be a scientist (or at least have a medical degree) to safely use peptides. This one always makes me smile because it's rooted in the intimidation women have felt for years when faced with anything scientific. You do not need to understand every chemical pathway to benefit from modern health tools. What matters is following reputable protocols, understanding basic safety guidelines, and listening to your body. The best peptide protocols are written in plain English, not code.

A third common misconception: "Peptides are just for men who want to get ripped." While it's true some bodybuilders use peptides for muscle gains, women's health clinics and longevity centers have made peptide therapy mainstream for everything from sleep support to skin renewal. If you look at clinics specializing in women's wellness, you'll see peptides recommended for issues like menopause symptoms, cognitive fog, chronic pain, and even libido. The stereotype that peptides are only about bulking up is outdated.

And yes, worries about effectiveness and safety are completely justified; after all, your health is precious. That's why I always lean on evidence, not hype. Research has shown that peptides like BPC-157 and CJC-1295 have low rates of serious side effects when used appropriately. Most side effects tend to be mild (think injection site redness or headache) and resolve with dose adjustments or stopping the product. Problems start when people buy from unregulated vendors or ignore dosing guidelines altogether, so vigilance matters.

Always ask for Certificates of Analysis from suppliers and look for providers who test their batches for purity.

It's easy to get swept up by influencer testimonials or before-and-after shots online. But spotting red flags is a skill worth building. As a general guideline, if a product promises unreasonably fast results or refuses to show third-party testing reports, just walk away. Be wary of sites with vague contact info or that push bundles without explaining what each peptide does. Even more concerning are so-called experts who discourage asking questions or who mock legitimate concerns about safety.

CHECKLIST
How to Vet a Peptide Claim or Product

- ✓ Does the provider list ingredients and batch numbers?
- ✓ Is there third-party lab testing available for purity?
- ✓ Are side effects and contraidications clearly explained?
- ✓ Does the protocol have references to reputable studies?
- ✓ Are customer reviews detailed and balanced—not just five-star raves?
- ✓ Can you contact real humans for support?

If you answer "no" to any of these, move on without guilt.

Feeling unsure is not a weakness, but wisdom in disguise. Skepticism means you want facts before you leap, and that is smart self-care. When talking to your doctor, frame peptide use as an informed health decision: "I've been researching peptide therapy for my energy levels and would love your thoughts on safety or interactions with my medications." If your partner expresses concern, try: "I'm exploring peptides because I want to feel better and have found protocols backed by reputable clinics and real studies." These conversations open doors instead of starting debates.

Peptide therapy isn't magic, but neither is it myth. It's a tool, one that deserves scrutiny and respect. As you keep reading, remember that curiosity paired with caution leads to confidence. You don't have to accept hype or fear as your only choices; with the right information, you can advocate for your health boldly and wisely.

TWO
GETTING STARTED WITH PEPTIDES: SAFETY, LEGALITY, AND SOURCING

IMAGINE FINALLY READYING YOURSELF TO TRY A PEPTIDE protocol after thorough research, only to hit a snag with a warning label: "For research use only. Not for human consumption." It's a common and valid concern—how legal is this purchase, and what are the risks if customs intervene? Many face this uncertainty, torn between eagerness and anxiety.

The legality of peptides is complex and depends on location, peptide type, and intended use. In the U.S., the FDA tightly regulates peptides; medical ones like insulin or certain weight-loss compounds require a prescription. Others occupy a "grey area", sold as "research chemicals" not intended for human use, but allowed for laboratory purposes. With a doctor's prescription at a compounding pharmacy, you're legally safe. However, ordering products labeled "not for human consumption" from research suppliers puts you in a legal grey area, as using these on yourself may technically break the law, even if widespread.

Canada is stricter. Most peptides require a prescription; unofficial purchases are illegal. Orders from abroad risk seizure, and importers may receive warnings about controlled substances. The

UK and EU generally follow a similar prescription model for medical use; peptides labeled for research can sometimes be obtained but not for self-administration. Each EU nation has its own nuances, but the approach is close to the UK's.

Australia has the toughest regulations: almost all peptides require a prescription, and importing without one is illegal. Border enforcement is strong, with even low-risk peptides tightly controlled.

	Region/Country	Prescription Only	Research-Use Only	OTC/Legal for Self-Use
	Prescription And Use Regulations By Region			
1	USA	Yes (most)	Yes (some)	Rare (insulin only)
2	Canada	Yes (most)	No	No
3	UK	Yes (some)	Yes	No
4	EU	Yes (varies)	Yes	No
5	Australia	Yes (all/most)	No	No

The key distinction is intent and labeling. Prescription peptides involve medical oversight. Those sold for research use are technically legal for labs but lack medical proofing and come without safety guarantees.

So, keep in mind that risks are real. One woman in California ordered BPC-157 from overseas, then watched her package get seized by customs, with only a letter notifying the violation. She lost her money and peace of mind; luckily, there were no legal charges. Other buyers have dealt with fraudulent charges or feared being flagged in databases. Even if unintentional, breaking regulations can result in fines or restrictions, and repeated offenses could escalate.

The safest way to access peptides is through licensed

compounding pharmacies, working with healthcare providers. Many doctors collaborate with specialty pharmacies to prepare custom peptide blends, providing documentation, dosing support, and assistance if problems arise. Start with your doctor or check local integrative medicine directories. Inquire if pharmacies are accredited (like the Pharmacy Compounding Accreditation Board in the U.S. or General Pharmaceutical Council in the UK) and confirm their sourcing from Good Manufacturing Practices (GMP) facilities.

Self-importation is risky; customs agents are trained to spot suspicious shipments, and laws change swiftly. Some attempt to use mail forwarders or disguise orders, but this gambles with both money and legal safety. Regulatory shifts occur as new studies or scandals emerge, making today's legal status uncertain tomorrow.

Key agencies to monitor include the FDA (US), MHRA (UK), EMA (EU), and TGA (Australia). These publish updates and warnings as laws change. Subscribing to their alerts is a proactive way to stay informed and will help avoid costly or stressful surprises.

Peptide Insights

Reflect on your reasons for considering peptides and the risks you're willing to take for potential benefits. Are you open to seeking a prescription, or would you prefer to wait for clearer regulations?

Write down your motivations and revisit them as your goals or the legal landscape evolves.

_____

_____

_____

_____

_____

_____

_____

_____

_____

_____

_____

Above all, aim to be well-informed and confident in your choices. The legal framework isn't meant to discourage, but to help you protect your health and finances as you pursue peptide therapy.

Vetting Peptide Sources

If you've ever felt a wave of anxiety when staring at a peptide supplier's website, you're not alone. It's overwhelming: endless options, shiny promises, and little clues about who to trust. The truth is, finding a safe and reliable source is half the battle. I always tell my clients that a little detective work upfront can spare you so much trouble later. You deserve transparency, and that starts with knowing exactly what to look for before you even think about clicking "add to cart."

First, begin with the basics: does the company clearly state who they are? Look for a physical address (not just a P.O. box), a working phone number, and direct email contact. A trustworthy supplier will list their business location including city, state, or country, and won't hide behind vague "contact us" forms. You should see lab certifications displayed openly: GMP (Good Manufacturing Practice) or ISO standards are gold. If they claim to use third-party labs, those labs should be named somewhere on their website. If anything is hidden or feels like a shell game, walk away. A reputable business wants you to know they're legitimate.

Transparency doesn't stop with the company's own site. Cross-check their reputation outside their own marketing bubble. Head to forums like Reddit's r/Biohackers, where users keep running lists of trusted and blacklisted suppliers—real people share actual experiences, both good and bad. Take time to scroll through recent threads; people will call out scams, share photos of real packaging, and update each other when suppliers change quality or practices. It's also worth checking review aggregators like Trustpilot or the Better Business Bureau. Look for patterns. For example, one bad review might be a fluke, but repeated complaints about "missing orders" or "no refunds" spell trouble. I like to hunt for consistent praise about customer service and quality; it's a good sign when long-time users vouch for a supplier.

When you reach out to a supplier with questions about products, ask for specifics: batch numbers, Certificates of Analysis (COAs), or detailed lab data. Pay attention to how they respond. If customer service gives vague answers, dances around your questions, or flat-out refuses to provide documentation, that's a bright red flag. Legitimate suppliers will send COAs without hesitation, as they want you to feel safe and confident in their products. Another warning: if they promise overnight shipping from overseas or insist on wire transfers only, be cautious. Fast shipping is nice, but not at the cost of safety or legality. Read refund policies with care; if they seem intentionally confusing or only offer store credit on defective items, consider it an alert.

Getting in the habit of documenting your process can protect you in case something goes sideways. I recommend starting with a small "test" order rather than going all-in on your first try. Choose the minimum quantity that still lets you inspect the product. Don't get upsold into buying more than you need for your initial experiment.

As soon as your order arrives, examine everything closely: packaging should be clean and professional, vials sealed, labels clear and matching what you ordered. Snap photos of everything (labels, seals, even shipping documents) so you have proof if there's a dispute. Keep all email correspondence with the supplier; a paper trail is your best ally if you need support or want to warn others.

Here's my **personal test order protocol**: I pick one product, usually the simplest formula available, and order it with tracked shipping. Once I receive it, I check expiration dates and batch numbers against the COA provided. If something doesn't match, such as a different number on the vial than on the report, don't use it and contact customer service immediately for an explanation. If the supplier makes excuses or drags things out, I treat it as a failed test and move on to another source.

It helps to think like an investigator: every supplier will claim purity and safety, but only the best will back up those claims when asked. If you ever feel pressured to buy quickly ("limited time sale!") or sense urgency from customer service reps in live chat boxes, pause and revisit your checklist. Patience here is protection.

For offline sources like compounding pharmacies, the same logic applies: ask for accreditations upfront and verify them with issuing bodies if possible. Don't hesitate to ask your pharmacist questions about sourcing or handling protocols; genuine professionals welcome informed clients who care about their health.

Use this checklist every time you explore a new supplier:

1. Does the company have a physical address and phone number?
2. Do they display lab certifications (GMP/ISO)?
3. Can they provide batch-specific COAs quickly?
4. Are they reviewed positively (and consistently) on third-party forums?
5. Does customer service answer questions directly and openly?
6. Is there a clear refund or replacement policy?
7. Are payment methods secure (credit card over wire transfer)?
8. Does packaging match online descriptions and arrive intact?

Document your answers before placing any order, and trust your instincts. If anything feels off or too good to be true, remember there are always other suppliers out there who value your safety as much as your business.

Reading Lab Reports to Ensure Purity and Avoid Scams

When you first see a Certificate of Analysis, or COA, it might look like a wall of numbers and technical jargon. But understanding how to read these reports is a powerful step in protecting yourself from scams and low-quality products. You deserve to know exactly what's going into your body. The COA acts as your behind-the-scenes pass, showing whether a peptide batch is pure, safe, and matches what the supplier promises. If you're new to this, start by looking for a few key fields: the batch or lot number, the peptide's name, the percentage of purity, the name of the testing lab, and the date the test was performed. Purity percentage is often front and center, and should be above 98% for any injectable peptide. Anything lower might mean unwanted byproducts, fillers, or even dangerous contaminants. I've seen COAs where the batch number on the report didn't match the number on the vial; that's a big red flag and usually signals someone reused a generic certificate for multiple products.

Lab names matter more than most people realize. Reputable COAs will come from independent third-party labs, not just an in-house company report. Look for details about the testing method used (like HPLC or mass spectrometry) and ask questions if you see vague language or missing data. Dates should be recent; if a COA is several years old, it's probably not valid for your batch. If you're ever presented with a blurry PDF or you notice obvious editing artifacts such as strange fonts, uneven lines, or missing elements, don't ignore your gut. Some sellers copy-and-paste text, hoping you won't notice small discrepancies. If you ever feel unsure, compare reports side by side for consistency. High-quality suppliers won't mind sharing these details because it shows they take your safety seriously.

Purity is important, especially for injectables. At 98% purity, you have confidence that only trace amounts of other substances are present. These traces generally pose no risk for healthy adults, but as purity drops toward 95% or below, risk increases. For oral peptides or beauty creams, slightly lower purity might be acceptable, but for anything entering your bloodstream, stick with the highest standard possible. Some companies try to impress buyers with 99.9% claims, but anything over 98% from a real lab is excellent. If purity isn't listed at all, or if the supplier can't show you a COA when you ask, that's your cue to find another source.

Also, note that the process of requesting a lab report should be transparent and simple. If you don't see a COA linked on the supplier's product page, it's completely appropriate to send a short, direct message like: "Hi, I'm interested in purchasing your BPC-157 peptide. Could you please provide a current Certificate of Analysis for the latest batch?" You don't have to explain yourself further; this is now standard practice among savvy buyers. If you get excuses like "We don't share that information," "It's proprietary," or "We'll send it after your purchase," thank them and move on. Your health is too important for mystery ingredients.

If you have any doubts about the document you receive, there are ways to double-check authenticity. You can send a small sample to an independent third-party testing lab (these can be found online with a quick search). Labs like Analytical Resource Labs or Eurofins will analyze your sample for identity and purity. This usually costs between $100 to $250 per test, which is a worthwhile investment if you're planning repeated use or large orders. These services give peace of mind and sometimes even catch suppliers who cut corners.

WHAT YOU'LL SEE ON A REAL COA

Batch Number:
Should match exactly with your vial or packaging.

Peptide Name:
Spelled out clearly; no abbreviations only.

Purity Percentage:
≥98% is gold standard

Testing Lab Name:
Must be independent

Test Date:
Preferably within the last year.

Testing Method:
HPLC or similar methods listed

Lab Contact Info:
Provides traceability

CERTIFICATE OF ANALYSIS

Batch Number:	123456
Peptide Name	ABC Peptide
Purity	≥98,0%
Testing Lab	Independent Lab
Test Date	2023-08-01
Method	HPLC
info@independentlab.com	

If any of this information is missing or looks suspicious, trust your instincts and don't use the product.

You might feel nervous about asking suppliers tough questions or requesting documentation—don't be! Every legitimate supplier expects it now. You're not being picky; you're being **smart and safe**. If you ever get stuck or aren't sure how to interpret a technical term on a COA, online communities are full of people who will happily help decode reports or flag concerns.

Understanding "Research Chemicals" vs. Prescription Peptides

If you've spent any time searching for peptides, you've most likely seen "research chemical" stamped across countless websites. This label isn't just a random marketing trick, it's a legal disclaimer meant to separate these products from anything a pharmacist might hand you with a doctor's note. When suppliers say "for research use only, not for human consumption," they're looking to shield themselves from legal trouble. They're essentially saying, "What you do with this is your business, not ours." The rules force them into this language, and as a customer, you need to know what that really means for your safety and rights.

So, what is a research chemical? In the peptide world, it's a compound sold for laboratory study or chemical experimentation (at least on paper). These are the vials and powders you find on sites with lots of disclaimers and little actual support. They're not produced in the same kind of tightly controlled facilities that prescription peptides are. There's no pharmacist double-checking the dose, no doctor overseeing your health, and no guarantee that the label matches the contents. Sometimes the product inside is perfectly pure and potent. Other times, it might be underdosed, contaminated, or even swapped out for something else entirely.

Prescription peptides live in a different category. These are made by regulated compounding pharmacies or pharmaceutical manufacturers under strict oversight. You need a licensed health provider to write a script, and the pharmacy prepares the product to those specifications. Quality control is built in; each batch is tested, and records are kept for every step. You get clear dosing instructions, access to professional follow-up, and confidence in what's going into your body. So, if something goes wrong, there's an accountability trail, and a real person with credentials who can answer your questions.

Comparing these two paths can feel like weighing convenience against peace of mind. Research chemicals offer easy online ordering, wide selection, and sometimes lower prices. The downside? Unpredictable quality and zero professional oversight. Prescription peptides require more effort (doctor appointments, paperwork, sometimes waiting lists), but they come with safety and consistency.

	Research Chemicals	Prescription Peptides
Sourcing	Online "research" vendors	Licensed pharmacies
Oversight	None	Medical professional required
Quality Control	Variable: COAs may be faked or reused	Strict batch testing; real COAs
Dosing	Not standardized: user must self-educate	Prescribed by provider
Cost	Often lower upfront	Higher (insurance may help)
Follow-up Support	None	Pharmacist and doctor on call
Legal Status	Gray area; disclaimers everywhere	Fully legal with prescription

Of course, risks with research chemicals go beyond just getting scammed.

Dosing can swing wildly even within the same brand, because there's so little oversight on how much active ingredient lands in each vial. I've seen reports from women who received two bottles of "the same" peptide; one did nothing, while the other caused unexpected side effects like headaches or swelling. Sometimes labels are switched at the packing stage or vials are filled with less than they claim. This implies so much more than money loss; it could mean you don't get results or, worse, you hurt yourself by taking too much or too little.

Mislabeled vials pose a particularly sneaky risk. Imagine mixing and injecting what you think is BPC-157 to help with recovery after an injury, only to realize later it was something else entirely, or a watered-down version that does nothing. With prescription peptides, every step is documented and traceable. Mistakes can happen anywhere in life, but they're much less likely when someone's license is on the line.

Deciding between research chemicals and prescription peptides really comes down to your goals, your comfort level with risk, and what's available where you live. If you need certainty (say you have a health condition or are especially sensitive to changes) working with a provider is the safer bet every time. If you're experimenting for wellness purposes, and feel comfortable doing your own vetting and monitoring, some people do choose research chemicals despite the risks.

Consider this quick decision tree: If your health concern is significant (chronic pain, recovery from surgery, hormone issues), prioritize safety by seeking a prescription route. If you're exploring peptides for mild wellness goals and understand both the legal grey area and how to vet suppliers thoroughly, research chemicals might be an option, but **always start low and go slow**. If you're uncomfortable with any uncertainty about what's in your vial or powder, don't compromise! Just wait until you can access peptides through legitimate medical channels.

No matter which route you take, stay informed and never hesitate to ask questions of suppliers, of your doctor, or of other women who have walked this path before you. Again, your wellbeing is worth more than any shortcut or bargain deal.

Spotting Safe vs. Risky Products

Nothing shakes your confidence more than holding a package you've waited weeks for, only to feel something is off. Spotting trouble before you inject or ingest anything is the kind of super-power you want in your wellness toolkit. If you're standing in your kitchen, turning a little vial over in your hands, and questioning whether it's safe, you're not alone. Let's talk about those red flags, the clues that should instantly slow you down or send you running.

Start with the packaging itself. If there's no lot number or batch code printed anywhere (whether on the vial, box, or label) that's a massive red flag. Legitimate products always track their batches for safety and recalls. Packaging that looks cheap or inconsistent (think blurry print, peeling stickers, or bottles that don't match the photos online) screams "corner-cutting." Sometimes, suppliers will use generic labels with nothing but a product name and "for research only", but if there's no lab data (like a batch-specific Certificate of Analysis) to back up what's in the bottle, you should be suspicious.

Another warning sign is price. If something costs half as much as every other source, you're likely not getting a deal, but being sold on desperation or trust. Peptide synthesis isn't cheap, and deep discounts usually mean diluted products or outright fakes.

Check how the product is sealed. If there's no tamper-evident seal like a snap-off cap or shrink wrap, you can't be sure what's happened since it left the factory. Inspect the solution inside (if it's a liquid): it should be clear, with no floating bits, cloudiness, or strange colors. Powdered peptides should look fine and uniform, never clumpy or discolored. Labels should be firmly attached, with professional printing and full details: product name (not just a code), strength or concentration, expiration date, storage instructions, the manufacturer's name, and ideally a QR code or batch reference. If any of these are missing, pause before going further.

The paperwork that comes with your shipment tells its own story. High-quality suppliers include a batch-specific Certificate of Analysis right in the box or provide a link to download it. This document proves that someone tested this specific batch for purity and identity. As we previously discussed, look for matching batch numbers between COA and vial; if they don't align, something's wrong. Professional labelling with sharp fonts and clear print without spelling errors often signals care at every step of production. Reliable products may even come with instructions for safe use and handling; extra points if there's a way to contact customer support printed on the box or paperwork.

When your package arrives, do a hands-on inspection before anything else. Open the package in good light and examine the color and consistency of any liquid or powder. Scan any QR codes to see if they link to actual documentation (not just a generic homepage).

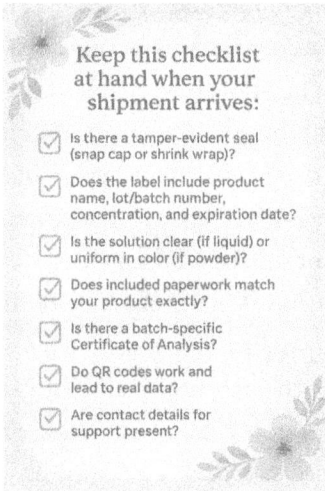

Keep this checklist at hand when your shipment arrives:

- ☑ Is there a tamper-evident seal (snap cap or shrink wrap)?
- ☑ Does the label include product name, lot/batch number, concentration, and expiration date?
- ☑ Is the solution clear (if liquid) or uniform in color (if powder)?
- ☑ Does included paperwork match your product exactly?
- ☑ Is there a batch-specific Certificate of Analysis?
- ☑ Do QR codes work and lead to real data?
- ☑ Are contact details for support present?

Read through any included paperwork. Does it match what you ordered? Take photos of everything for your records before opening or mixing anything. If you spot anything suspicious like missing labels, broken seals, cloudy solutions, mismatched paperwork, or QR codes that go nowhere, STOP immediately.

If you find yourself holding a suspicious product, don't panic but act quickly. First, take detailed photos of every part of the packaging and product. Contact the supplier right away with your concerns; sometimes mistakes happen in packing and can be fixed quickly. If they refuse to address your questions or offer vague excuses ("That's just how it comes," "No one else has complained"), escalate your response. Report unsafe products to consumer watchdog groups like the Better Business Bureau or FDA MedWatch (in the US). In other countries, look for medicine safety authorities who handle supplement fraud. Never dispose of questionable peptides in household trash or pour them down the drain; most pharmacies will accept them for safe disposal as biohazardous materials.

Reporting helps shield others from falling into the same trap.

If you encounter a scammy supplier or dangerous product, please share your experience on community forums so others know what to avoid. Your vigilance and voice are powerful tools in making this space safer for everyone searching for their best health.

Talking to Healthcare Providers about Peptide Use

It's common to feel nervous about discussing peptides with your doctor, especially if you fear skepticism. Being prepared helps: honestly share your goals ("I'm looking for safer options for energy and recovery and want your input"), which sets a tone of respect and collaboration.

If your provider is hesitant or unfamiliar, guide the discussion: "I know peptides aren't mainstream, but I've read promising studies and want to be safe. Could you review a protocol with me?" With open providers, be more specific: "I'm considering BPC-157 for injury recovery, using this dosing protocol. Is there anything in my history I should watch for?" For skeptical providers, stay factual: if they mention lack of evidence, you can reply, "I understand your caution. I've brought some recent studies and a Certificate of Analysis. Would you look these over so we can decide together?" Emphasize a collaborative approach—focus on working together, not convincing.

Pharmacists can also help: "I'm starting peptide therapy and want to check for interactions with my current meds. Can we review my list?" OB/GYNs may know less about peptides but know hormones well, so try, "Since I'm managing perimenopause, I'm exploring peptides for support. Have any of your patients tried this? Any safety concerns for someone like me?"

Present research as a starting point for discussion, not instruction. Hand your provider a summary or COA: "Here's what I found. Can you help interpret this or flag issues?"

If you sense resistance, don't push, just ask if they'd look into it and suggest following up at your next visit.

Explaining Protocols, Research, and Safety Measures

You will build trust quickly by showing you're prepared. Bring a one-page summary: peptide name, dosing plan, intended benefits, and monitoring strategy. For example: "I'll use BPC-157 at 250 mcg daily for four weeks, then reassess. This clinical paper guided my plan." Highlight key findings or safety notes to save your provider from sifting through long articles.

Clearly outline how you'll monitor for side effects: "I'll track bloodwork (liver, kidney) monthly, watch for symptoms, and record how I feel. If something seems wrong, I'll stop and contact you." Share your tracking system (an app or journal) and invite input, as providers may notice gaps you missed.

When sharing research, provide only peer-reviewed studies or official safety data. Avoid blog posts or influencer content. Attach a Certificate of Analysis for your peptide if possible, saying, "This shows batch purity and independent testing." Ask for input on any possible gaps or concerns regarding your plan.

Handling Objections and Documenting Decisions

Providers typically raise **three main concerns**: legality, lack of FDA approval, and safety.

If told, "These aren't FDA approved," agree and add, "That's why I want your guidance." If they raise safety: "That's exactly why I'm coming to you first." For legality: "I'm sourcing from a compounding pharmacy and have checked the regulations as best as I can."

If your provider remains unwilling, you can ask if they'll document your discussion for your medical record, as this adds accountability and future reference.

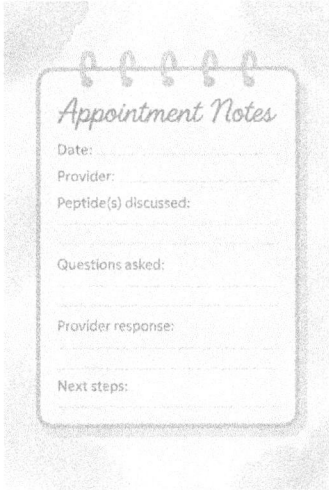

Appointment Notes

Date:

Provider:

Peptide(s) discussed:

Questions asked:

Provider response:

Next steps:

Take notes during your appointment: date, what was discussed, advice given, and next steps. This documentation keeps everyone aligned and gives peace of mind if issues arise.

Conversation Starters

- "I've researched this peptide's safety. Could you help interpret the findings?"
- "How does this protocol fit with my current medications?"
- "What monitoring precautions do you recommend?"

Prepared, open-minded conversations show respect for your provider's expertise while taking responsibility for your health, a balance that often leads to greater trust—even from skeptical providers.

The main takeaway here is that safety starts with open communication, both with yourself and your care team. Clear, respectful self-advocacy makes every step steadier.

THREE

THE ART AND SCIENCE OF PEPTIDE PROTOCOLS

STANDING IN FRONT OF YOUR BATHROOM MIRROR, toothbrush in hand, you stare at your reflection like it owes you an apology. You've had it with the endless promises of wellness magic. You're not asking for a miracle, just the ability to wake up feeling human, move without sounding like a creaky door, or maybe, just maybe, see your skin look like it's been on a spa vacation. What you need is an approach that actually *gets you*, not another one-size-fits-all solution. Enter your personal peptide protocol. A real game plan for real results, not more 'wellness confusion' to add to the pile."

Building your protocol starts with defining a real, personal goal, rather than just picking a random peptide or copying advice from a stranger online.

What would truly make you feel better?

Is it enough energy to finish the workday without an afternoon slump?

Losing five stubborn pounds after a tough year?

Healing lingering tendon pain that's keeping you from yoga?

Or seeing smoother, more radiant skin in the morning?

The more specific your goal, the easier it is to measure progress and success. Avoid vague intentions like "feel better"—anchor your biohacking to something tangible.

I recommend using the SMART framework: Specific, Measurable, Achievable, Relevant, and Time-bound. Instead of "I want to lose weight," try "I want to lose 7 pounds in 8 weeks and have the energy to play with my kids after dinner." If healing is your target: "Lower my tennis elbow pain from 6 to below 3 within four weeks of peptide therapy." Skin goals? "Improve skin texture and reduce fine lines around my eyes in 12 weeks." Clearly defined goals help you recognize whether your protocol is making a difference, and let you pivot if needed.

Once your goal is set, choosing a peptide becomes much simpler. Every peptide has a unique superpower backed by research and real-world results. For example, if you're healing an injury, BPC-157 is well-regarded for soft-tissue repair and decreasing inflammation. For stubborn fat, CJC-1295 encourages natural growth hormone, supporting fat loss and muscle preservation. GHK-Cu is popular for skin, thanks to its collagen-boosting and rejuvenation effects. For mind support, Selank gently promotes calm and mental clarity.

Goal	Best Peptide(s)	Primary Effect
Injury Repair	BPC-157	Aids tendon/ligament healing
Fat Loss	CJC-1295	Boosts growth hormone for fat loss
Skin Rejuvenation	GHK-Cu	Boosts collagen, improves elasticity
Cognitive Boost	Selank	Calms anxiety, enhances mental clarity
Muscle Recovery	TB-500	Improves muscle regeneration

It's best to start with just one goal and one peptide. Although tempting to stack multiple peptides, beginning simple is safest and will give you clarity on what's actually working. Focus on a single change, and expand only once you recognize results or feel ready.

Before starting, gather baseline measurements.

- For fat loss: record your weight or body measurements (waist, hips).
- For pain: track daily or weekly discomfort on a 1–10 scale.
- Skin improvements: take a well-lit "before" photo and note concerns like texture or fine lines.

These tracking methods provide honest feedback and help spot even subtle changes. And remember, selecting peptides for your health isn't about chasing the trendiest option, but understanding what's most important to you, aligning scientific evidence with your goals, and moving forward step by step.

Protocol Mapping Worksheet

This following list will help to map your first protocol:

1. My Primary Goal:
(e.g., "Heal right shoulder pain from 7/10 to under 3/10 in 6 weeks.")

2. Chosen Peptide:
(e.g., BPC-157)

3. Baseline Measurement:
(e.g., Pain at 7/10; limited overhead reach)

4. Protocol Start Date:
(e.g., May 1st)

5. Intended Outcome & Timeline:
(e.g., Pain down to 3/10, regain full reach by June 12th)

6. Tracking Method:
(Daily pain scores, weekly shoulder movement videos)

7. Any Other Notes:
(Current meds, supplements, allergies, previous therapies)

Dosage Demystified: Finding the Right Amount for Your Body

When you're staring at a tiny vial of peptide and a stack of instructions, it's easy to feel a little nervous. Dosage talk online can get overwhelming fast, full of numbers, units, and wild claims. You might see mcg, mg, or even IU and wonder, "How much is actually right for me?"

Let's take the confusion out of it. The smartest way to start is always "low and slow." Your body is unique: your size, metabolism, sensitivity, and even stress levels shape how you'll respond. You don't want to dump a huge dose in your system and hope for the best. Instead, you want to nudge your body, watch how it reacts, and only increase the dose if needed.

Most peptides are measured in micrograms (mcg) or milligrams (mg). For a quick reference: 1 mg equals 1,000 mcg. Some peptides, like CJC-1295, are dosed between 100–300 mcg per injection for women. BPC-157 for injury repair often falls in the 250–500 mcg per day range. If you ever see IUs (international units), those usually appear with growth hormone or insulin-related peptides.

The "start low, go slow" ladder is a reliable and safe method. Imagine a ladder with rungs labeled 100 mcg, 200 mcg, 300 mcg. Begin on the first rung for a week or two, watch your body's signals, and only step up if you're not seeing results and feel good. Sometimes the lowest dose is all you need. Pushing higher without reason can lead to side effects or wasted product.

Personalizing will involve looking at your weight, age, and how your body usually responds to new things. Lighter women or those who are sensitive to medications often need lower starting doses. Here's how you'd do the math: If BPC-157 recommends 2–4 mcg per kg of body weight daily, and you weigh 140 lbs (about 64 kg), your range is 128–256 mcg daily. Most women settle in the middle and adjust based on what they feel. If you're over 50 or have health issues, start at the lower end.

Dosing frequency matters too. Some peptides need daily injections, whereas others might call for a few times a week. Always read the label and protocol carefully.

Most peptides are injected in very small volumes, often 0.2 ml or less, using insulin syringes that make it easy to measure out precise amounts. When you get your peptide as powder in a vial, you'll need to reconstitute it with bacteriostatic water before drawing doses. For example, if you have a 5 mg vial and add 2 ml water, each 0.1 ml equals 250 mcg. Drawing up the dose means gently tilting the vial, inserting the needle through the rubber stopper, and slowly pulling back until the plunger lines up with your target mark. If air bubbles sneak in, tap them out gently before injecting.

If you're using reconstituting powder, always wash your hands first, use a fresh alcohol pad on the vial top, and let the water run down the side of the vial to avoid frothing up the powder. Swirl gently; don't shake hard or you'll damage the peptide chains. Keep the vial in the fridge between uses to preserve potency.

Knowing when you've found your "sweet spot" dose comes from tracking both how you feel and any visible changes.

Underdosing often means no change or progress stalls: pain lingers, skin stays dull, or energy doesn't budge.

Overdosing might show up as headaches, swelling at injection sites, nausea, or feeling jittery or wired.

The **best dose** is where you get steady benefits, like less pain or better sleep, without weird side effects.

Symptom Checklist: *Is Your Dose Right?*

- Energy level (1–10): Has it improved after one week?
- Sleep quality: Falling asleep faster? Staying asleep?
- Pain or injury: Noticeable drop in pain scores?
- Skin: Smoother texture or fewer breakouts?
- Mood and focus: Any boost or stability?
- Side effects: Any nausea, headaches, swelling?

Jot these answers down each week. Patterns will jump out faster than you expect.

Don't forget, everybody's chemistry is different. If you hit side effects, drop your dose back down or pause for a few days before trying again at half-strength. Always give yourself time. **Peptides work in cycles**, not overnight miracles. If nothing changes after three weeks at a moderate dose and your supplier checks out, it may be time to tweak your protocol or consult with a healthcare provider.

Above all, trust yourself and your body's feedback more than any internet dosing chart. **Start small, listen closely, adjust patiently**.

Timing and Cycling: Maximize Results and Minimize Risks

When you're starting with peptides, it's easy to get caught up in the "what" and "how much" and forget about the "when." Yet timing can honestly make or break your results. Your body isn't a robot; hormones, digestion, and even your sleep-wake cycles all shape how well a peptide works.

For instance, if you're using CJC-1295 to support fat loss or muscle recovery, research and real-world reports agree: take it at night before bed, ideally on an empty stomach. This lines up with your body's natural growth hormone release, which peaks during deep sleep. Eating a meal too close to your dose, especially if it's full of carbs, can blunt the effect since insulin competes with growth hormone. BPC-157, often chosen for injury recovery, works best when taken at roughly the same time each day, but you don't have to stress about fasting or bedtime—just aim for consistency. For acute injuries, some women split the dose, taking half in the morning and half at night to keep healing signals steady.

Here's a simple reference table you can use:

Peptide	Best Timing	Notes
CJC-1295	Night, pre-sleep	Empty stomach; avoid food 1-2 hours
BPC-157	Any, consistent	Split AM/PM for injury recovery
GHK-Cu	Morning	Topically after cleansing skin
Selank	Morning or as needed	For mood/focus; can be flexible

Now, let's talk cycles. Cycling peptides means you're not taking them 24/7, 365 days a year. Your body needs time to reset its receptors. That's how you avoid building up tolerance (called downregulation), which happens when your cells start ignoring the peptide's message after too much exposure. Breaks also give you space to reflect on progress and catch subtle side effects before they become problems.

A classic cycle is "5 days on, 2 days off" each week, which mimics the body's natural need for rest and lets you see how you feel on both "on" and "off" days. For longer-running protocols, an 8-week stint followed by 4 weeks off is common, especially with peptides like CJC-1295 or TB-500. You'll want to mark this out on your calendar the way you would a round of antibiotics or a fitness challenge.

Think of a visual timeline: Week 1 through Week 8 marked in green (active peptide days), then Weeks 9 through 12 in blue (rest/recovery). This gives your body a pause and lets you evaluate whether the protocol is still working or needs tweaking. If you notice your results stalling, like weight loss slowing down or injury healing plateauing, a cycle break is usually the fix. Receptors "reset" during time off, making the next round more effective. Signs that it's time for a break include results flatlining, new side effects popping up (like swelling or fatigue), or just a gut sense that something feels off.

Logging when you take **each dose and cycle** makes troubleshooting so much easier down the line. You can use a simple journal, a notes app on your phone, or even a printable calendar you hang on the fridge. Note the day and time of each dose, symptoms, mood, energy, sleep quality, and any changes in pain or skin. If you're cycling peptides for several weeks at a stretch, jot down mid-cycle check-ins: "Week 4: Energy up, pain down from 7 to 4." When you hit your off-cycle weeks, note any rebound effects, cravings, or fatigue.

Sample Cycle Log

Date: _____

Peptide: _____

Dose: _____

Time taken: _____

Mood/energy (1–10): _____

Pain/skin/focus (score): ____

Any side effects?: _____

Cycle week: _____

This log is deigned to become your safety net if something goes sideways or if you need to share your experience with a doctor or online support group. Over time, these logs reveal patterns, like if sleep improves most during weeks 2–4 or if mild headaches always show up on day six of your cycle. You'll start to spot your body's rhythms and know exactly when it's time to rest or adjust.

Cycling helps avoid tolerance while treating your body with respect and listening as it changes week by week. Sometimes you'll feel fantastic two weeks in and want to keep going forever; other times, life throws curveballs like travel, illness, or stress that call for pausing early. There's no shame in adjusting for real life. If you're not seeing results by the end of a cycle, review your log for missed doses, poor timing (like late-night snacks with CJC-1295), or signs that you might need a different peptide altogether.

Stacking Peptides

Stacking is a term you'll hear tossed around a lot in peptide circles, and it simply means using more than one peptide at the same time to get a stronger or broader effect.

For some, stacking can feel like building a wellness recipe, each ingredient with a purpose, supporting your bigger picture. The trick is knowing when to add that second or third peptide, and when to hold back. You want to be sure you truly understand how your body responds to one peptide before layering in another. I always tell my clients: get comfortable with the basics before you start mixing. If you've never used peptides before, stick with just one for at least a full cycle. For instance, try BPC-157 alone if you're aiming to heal a nagging joint or tendon. Watch for real changes in pain, swelling, or range of motion. Once you're confident it's working (or not), only then consider adding something like TB-500 for more stubborn, chronic injuries.

You might be wondering if there are stacks specially designed for women's most common goals. The answer is yes, and these are the ones I see helping women the most, both in research and real-world results. For fat loss, a classic stack pairs CJC-1295 with Ipamorelin. This duo works by nudging your natural growth hormone release without suppressing your own hormone production, which is especially important for women who want to avoid harsh side effects. The protocol usually looks like this: CJC-1295 and Ipamorelin both injected before bed, five nights a week, cycling off after eight weeks for a rest period. Women often report better sleep, easier fat loss (especially around the midsection), and improved muscle tone, all without feeling "wired" or jittery.

If radiant skin tops your wishlist, there's a stack that combines GHK-Cu (a copper peptide) with Thymosin Beta-4. GHK-Cu targets skin elasticity and collagen production, so fine lines and dullness start to fade. Thymosin Beta-4 steps in to accelerate healing and reduce inflammation, which can help with redness, acne scars, or slow-to-heal spots. These two are often used together as a topical serum at night, sometimes with an injectable form of Thymosin Beta-4 for those dealing with bigger skin concerns or scarring. For perimenopause or hormone swings, stacking CJC-1295 with KISS-1 has shown promise. KISS-1 signals the body to balance reproductive hormones more naturally, which can stabilize mood and cycle irregularities without synthetic hormones.

The secret to effective stacking isn't just throwing peptides together, but sequencing and scheduling so they don't trip each other up or overload your system. You'll want to stagger injection times if you're using more than one injectable peptide. CJC-1295 and Ipamorelin can be taken together at night, but if you add BPC-157 for injury repair, it's better to take that in the morning or early evening so your body isn't processing everything at once. For topical stacks like GHK-Cu plus Thymosin Beta-4, apply them one after another instead of blending together; this way, each peptide absorbs fully before the next goes on.

Troubleshooting a stack takes patience and a bit of detective work. Sometimes your body will react in unexpected ways (a sudden headache, new skin irritation, or sleep disruption) and you'll wonder which peptide is the culprit. The best move is to pause all but one peptide and give your body three to five days to adjust. If symptoms clear up, reintroduce one peptide at a time every three days while tracking how you feel. This stepwise approach will quickly isolate the source of any issue.

Stacks aren't forever. Use them strategically, perhaps a few weeks for fat loss before a big event, or a skin stack during winter months when dryness flares up. Always cycle off for at least as long as you were on, giving your body time to recalibrate. This respect for rhythm helps minimize risk while maximizing your results.

Key Takeaways...

Timing is Everything: For peptides like CJC-1295, timing your dose is key. Take it before bed, ideally on an empty stomach, to align with your body's natural growth hormone cycle.

Consistency is Key: BPC-157 is all about routine. Take it at the same time daily, and for injury recovery, consider splitting your dose for steady healing.

Cycling Peptides: Don't use peptides nonstop! Giving your body a break (like the classic "5 days on, 2 days off" routine) helps prevent tolerance and ensures you're actually benefiting from the protocol.

Track Your Progress: Keep a log of your doses, symptoms, and changes, whether it's better sleep, improved energy, or healing. This way, you can adjust based on real feedback.

Stacking: Start simple. Master one peptide before adding another to avoid overwhelming your system. Stagger injections and always track your body's responses for any unexpected side effects.

. . .

Take It Slow: Peptide stacking isn't a race. Go slow, experiment safely, and trust your body's feedback. Less is often more, especially when you're aiming for long-term results over quick fixes.

Sub-Q, IM, and Oral: Choosing the Best Delivery Method

How you take your peptide significantly affects both your results and comfort. Peptides usually aren't effective when swallowed like vitamins because stomach acid breaks them down. That's why subcutaneous (sub-Q) and intramuscular (IM) injections are so common. Sub-Q injections are suitable for at-home use. They deliver peptides just beneath the skin into the fat layer using tiny, insulin-like needles, and are generally less painful and easier for beginners. IM injections go deeper, directly into muscle tissue (like the outer thigh or upper arm), requiring longer needles and often causing more discomfort. While IM works for some peptides, sub-Q is typically more approachable.

Recently, oral and nasal delivery methods have grown in popularity, especially among women who dislike needles or have trouble with injecting. As previously mentioned, these means aren't as effective for all peptides due to digestive enzymes breaking down many oral forms before they're absorbed. However, drugs like Selank are just as effective as injections when given as a nasal spray.

For beginners, sub-Q is often the best blend of safety, ease, and effectiveness.

Before injecting, wash your hands thoroughly, clean the injection site (commonly lower abdomen, about two inches from your belly button) with an alcohol pad, and let it dry.

Draw up your dose with a fresh insulin syringe, making sure to remove any air bubbles.

Pinch a small fold of skin, hold the syringe like a pencil at a 45-degree angle, insert swiftly, push the plunger, and withdraw.

Dab with a tissue if you see a drop of blood. Initial nerves are normal, but most people find the process easier and less painful than expected.

You can alternate injection spots between the lower abdomen, outer thigh, or upper hip (flank) to avoid irritation. To help ensure rotation, imagine a tic-tac-toe grid on your abdomen and move to a new square each time. Avoid injecting into sore or bruised skin, and always use a new sterile needle to prevent infection and reduce pain and bruising. Never reuse needles. If you notice redness or pain that lasts more than 48 hours, consult a healthcare professional. Keep a simple log or calendar to track your injection sites.

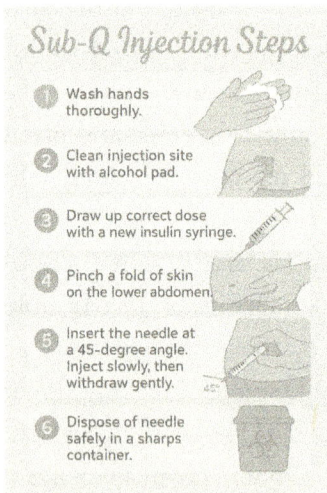

Sub-Q Injection Steps

1 Wash hands thoroughly.

2 Clean injection site with alcohol pad.

3 Draw up correct dose with a new insulin syringe.

4 Pinch a fold of skin on the lower abdomen.

5 Insert the needle at a 45-degree angle. Inject slowly, then withdraw gently.

6 Dispose of needle safely in a sharps container.

Needle-free options like nasal sprays are effective for select peptides, particularly for mood, sleep, or cognitive benefits. Selank nasal spray, for example, is simple to use; just follow dosing instructions, typically administered in the morning or as needed. Oral peptides such as collagen or new gut health formulations can be taken as powders or capsules, but may require higher, more expensive doses for comparable results since digestion destroys much of the peptide.

If you're uncomfortable or squeamish with needles but still want injectable peptides, ask a nurse, friend, or watch reliable online tutorials to help build confidence. Practicing with an empty syringe on an orange can also ease fears.

Choosing the delivery method that's right for you is just as important as picking the right peptide. Safety, comfort, and sustainability for your daily routine should come first.

If you're uncertain or make a mistake, don't hesitate to pause, review instructions, or ask someone experienced for guidance. The process should be safe, effective, and something you feel comfortable maintaining. Women deserve options that fit their bodies and comfort zones.

Protocols: Plug-and-Play Routines for Beginners

Starting with peptides can feel overwhelming, but having a clear routine makes all the difference. Playbooks offer simple, structured protocols you can follow, helping you track progress and avoid second-guessing. With these routines, it's easier to stay consistent and see measurable results.

For **fat loss**, beginners often use CJC-1295 and Ipamorelin. Inject both peptides subcutaneously before bed, five nights per week, for 8 weeks. Standard doses range from 100–200 mcg each (always check your vial and instructions). Avoid eating for at least 90 minutes before the injection, as insulin can reduce effectiveness. Set reminders, mark your calendar, and track your morning energy, appetite, and sleep quality. Weigh yourself and note body measurements every week. After eight weeks, take a break of 2–4 weeks before considering another cycle.

For **skin rejuvenation**, apply a GHK-Cu topical serum nightly after cleansing. Massage a small amount into target areas such as around the eyes or dull cheeks. For extra healing, add oral BPC-157 (250 mcg daily). These steps often yield a healthier glow in the first month, with more noticeable changes by week eight. Take before-and-after photos every four weeks and look for improvements in skin tone and firmness.

Injury recovery is a key area for peptides. Use BPC-157 (250–500 mcg) as a daily sub-Q injection near the injury for 4–6 weeks. Log pain on a scale of one to ten and note any improvement in daily movements. Reassess after four weeks; if there's no progress, consider pausing or adjusting your approach.

For **mood or stress support**, Selank nasal spray may help. Use two sprays (100 mcg each) in the morning or when calm focus is needed, such as before work or during stressful moments. Many users notice effects quickly—check in with yourself by evening, and again after a week. Note changes in tension, mood, and focus.

Tracking and safety are crucial, so please use a daily checklist:

- Did you take your dose?
- Any side effects?
- How was your energy?

Each week, review your log for patterns such as improvements in sleep, pain, or other symptoms. Spend a few minutes every Sunday to check your progress, perhaps also taking photos or measurements, depending on your goals.

· · ·

Routines aren't always perfect. Life gets busy, and sometimes you might miss a dose or feel injection site soreness. If you skip a dose, simply resume the schedule, and never double up. For mild redness or swelling, rotate injection sites and use a cold compress. If discomfort lasts over 48 hours or seems unusual, contact your healthcare provider.

Be patient. Progress can take three to four weeks, and plateaus or ups and downs are likely to occur. If you see no improvement in six weeks, review your logs for consistency or other routine changes. Sometimes adjusting dose timing or improving sleep is enough to get back on track.

_____

_____

_____

_____

_____

_____

_____

_____

_____

_____

_____

Protocol Customization Worksheet

Protocol Name:
(*What is the name of the peptide protocol you're starting?*)

Start Date:
(*When will you begin this protocol?*)

<u>Daily Goal/Checklist</u>

☐ **Morning:**
(*List the peptides or supplements to take in the morning.*)

☐ **Afternoon:**
(*List the peptides or supplements to take in the afternoon.*)

☐ **Evening:**
(*List the peptides or supplements to take in the evening.*)

☐ **Hydration:**
(*Track your daily water intake.*)

☐ **Exercise:**
(*Write down your daily exercise routine.*)

☐ **Sleep Goals:**
(*Note your target sleep duration or sleep habits for the day.*)

<u>Weekly Review</u>

Week Starting:
(*Start date of your week for review.*)

Energy Level (1-10):
(*Rate your overall energy level from 1 to 10.*)

Sleep Quality (1-10):
(*Rate your sleep quality from 1 to 10.*)

Mood (1-10):

(*Rate your mood from 1 to 10.*)

Physical Changes:

(*Note any physical changes, improvements, or challenges you've noticed.*)

Peptide Effectiveness:

(*How well do you feel the peptide protocol is working for you?*)

Adjustments to Make:

(*List any adjustments needed in dosage, timing, or any other aspect.*)

Monthly Progress Photo/Measurement

Date of Photo/Measurement:

(*Note the date for your photo/measurement updates.*)

Photo:

(*Take a progress photo from the front, side, and back.*)

Weight/Body Measurements:

(*Take your weight and body measurements for comparison.*)

Skin/Appearance Changes:

(*Note any changes in your skin, hair, nails, etc.*)

Notes & Adjustments

Jot down thoughts, challenges, or additional changes to consider for the next phase of your protocol. Any new observations or side effects can also go here.

FOUR

PEPTIDE BIOHACKS FOR ENERGY, FAT LOSS, AND METABOLISM

WE'VE ALL FACED MORNINGS WHEN HITTING SNOOZE FEELS unavoidable and the day's demands seem overwhelming. Many women want a steady, natural energy boost, something beyond caffeine's temporary lift, which often leads to jitters and crashes. What most of us seek is deeper, more sustainable vitality: a way to genuinely support cellular energy. Peptides offer this solution.

MOTS-c is a small peptide that acts inside your cells' mitochondria, the "powerhouses" of your body. This peptide improves how cells use glucose while enhancing fat burning, promoting lasting alertness and resilience instead of short-lived stimulation. Unlike conventional quick fixes, MOTS-c collaborates with your metabolism to sustain stamina and curb mid-afternoon slumps. Many women who try it notice steadier energy all day and better workout performance, especially if light activity usually leaves them tired or if energy drops as the day goes on.

Another effective approach is the CJC-1295 and Ipamorelin stack. Together, these peptides nudge your body to make more natural growth hormone. This is not at extreme, bodybuilder levels, but enough to help you recover quicker, sleep deeper, and wake up refreshed. CJC-1295 provides a gentle, extended hormone release, while Ipamorelin gives a brief, clean pulse without affecting other hormones like cortisol or prolactin. Women who use this combo frequently report better mental focus, mood, and stable energy.

You should know that fitting these protocols into a busy life doesn't have to be complicated. For MOTS-c, the optimal schedule is a subcutaneous injection in the morning, just after waking and before breakfast. Pair this with ten minutes of early sunlight exposure to reset your circadian rhythm; it's an easy habit that maximizes MOTS-c's benefits. CJC-1295/Ipamorelin are injected together after your last meal, syncing with your natural sleep-related growth hormone surge so you wake up feeling renewed.

If daily life is packed with nonstop meetings or late nights, here's a practical routine: inject MOTS-c upon waking (even if you rely on coffee) followed by a glass of water and a few deep breaths by a window. Save the CJC-1295/Ipamorelin dose for bedtime to avoid daytime drowsiness.

Combining peptides with a variety of simple biohacks amplifies results without overstimulating your system. Quick morning sunlight (ten minutes after you get up) helps regulate cortisol and smooths your energy curve. Cold exposure, like 30 seconds of cold water at the end of your shower, further boosts alertness, particularly when paired with MOTS-c. For added stress resilience, try adaptogens like rhodiola or ashwagandha in the morning; these herbs buffer stress and prevent energy crashes without stimulants' jittery effects. If you feel overamped after starting peptides, cut back on adaptogens and make sure you're including slow carbs at breakfast.

Common mistakes with energy peptides stem from overuse or ignoring signs from your body's sleep patterns. Trouble falling asleep or odd nighttime wakings may mean you're dosing MOTS-c too late or using too much CJC-1295/Ipamorelin. Too much evening energy can signal overdosing or poor timing. Warning signs like irritability, racing thoughts, or feeling both "wired and tired" suggest you should pause or decrease dosage. Moreover, never compromise sleep for energy; deep rest is essential for peptides to work effectively.

Peptide Insights

Time to pause and ponder. How does your energy fluctuate during a typical week?

Spend a few minutes noting when you feel most alert and when fatigue hits. Write down factors that might influence these trends, such as sleep, meals, or stressors. Use these notes as a baseline before starting any peptide protocol to track real changes.

_____

_____

_____

_____

_____

_____

_____

_____

_____

_____

_____

Fat Loss Protocols

Most women who reach out about fat loss are already tired of quick fixes and empty promises. You want results that respect your hormones, protect your muscle, and truly last.

Here's where peptides like CJC-1295 and Ipamorelin step into the spotlight. These peptides don't burn fat with a sledgehammer; they tap into your body's own messaging system. Simply put, CJC-1295 mimics a natural hormone that signals your pituitary gland to release growth hormone in pulses—never flooding your body, but giving you gentle surges, especially at night. Growth hormone makes fat cells break down their stores, a process called lipolysis. It's like flipping a switch so your body accesses fat for energy, not just carbohydrates. Ipamorelin complements CJC-1295 by triggering a similar pulse but without spiking hunger or messing with cortisol, which means you get the benefits without feeling ravenous or stressed out. For women, this stack is attractive because it preserves lean muscle and helps you lose the right kind of weight: actual fat, not precious muscle mass or water.

Neither CJC-1295 nor Ipamorelin disrupts estrogen or progesterone directly, so you don't have to worry about wild mood swings or period chaos from the peptides alone. Still, because growth hormone nudges your metabolism, it's smart to start with a conservative dose and work your way up only if you tolerate it well. Most studies and clinical practices recommend 100 micrograms of each peptide, injected subcutaneously, five nights per week. For best results, inject at least two hours after your last meal, right before bed. This timing lines up with your body's natural hormone rhythms.

The "8-Week Fat Loss Accelerator" protocol is something I've seen work for many women who want structure and steady progress. For eight weeks, you'll inject 100mcg CJC-1295 plus 100mcg Ipamorelin subcutaneously, five nights a week (Monday to

Friday works for most). Take weekends off to let your receptors reset; a little break keeps results coming and lowers the chance of side effects. After eight weeks, pause for at least four weeks before starting another cycle. During this break, continue tracking your food and exercise; you'll likely notice your metabolism stays higher for weeks after stopping.

To **amplify your results**, pair this protocol with a high-protein, moderate-carb diet. Aim for protein at every meal (chicken, fish, Greek yogurt, eggs) because growth hormone works best when your body has the building blocks to repair and maintain muscle. Don't ditch carbs entirely; whole grains and sweet potatoes support recovery and will keep you from feeling depleted. Also, on peptide cycles, strength training is your best friend. Focus on compound lifts such as squats, deadlifts, push-ups, or even resistance bands if you're new to weights. Two to three days a week is enough to make a difference. If possible, mix in one or two sessions of HIIT (high intensity interval training), as short bursts of effort spike growth hormone naturally and maximize fat burning.

Cycles matter, particularly for women's bodies. If you're premenopausal with regular periods, keep an eye on how you feel during the luteal phase (the two weeks before your period). Water retention usually spikes here thanks to progesterone shifts, so it's normal to see the scale climb or cravings increase. Don't panic or ramp up your dose. Instead, use that week for gentle movement like walking or yoga. If you feel puffy or tired, add magnesium-rich foods and hydrate more; this helps flush excess water and supports muscle relaxation. For women in perimenopause or post-menopause, fat can settle stubbornly around the belly due to dropping estrogen. Peptides will help shift your metabolism back in your favor, especially if you combine the protocol with regular resistance training and avoid crash diets.

If you're postmenopausal and feel like nothing moves the needle anymore, start with the lowest dose possible (even half:

50mcg CJC-1295 + 50mcg Ipamorelin) for the first two weeks, then increase if you tolerate it well. Your recovery time may be longer than in your thirties or forties. Give yourself grace and measure progress with photos, tape measures, or how your clothes fit, rather than just the scale.

Women sometimes ask if they should adjust dosing during their period or skip injections when traveling or sick. I say, listen to your body above all else. If you're run down or fighting an infection, it's okay to pause for several days, and resuming when you feel better won't erase your progress.

Metabolic Reset

If you're frustrated by constant cravings, unpredictable appetite, or sluggish metabolism, you're not alone. Many of us experience shifts in hunger cues after thirty and struggle with blood sugar swings that leave us tired and irritable.

GLP-1 agonists like semaglutide and liraglutide offer a peptide-based approach to reset appetite, enhance insulin sensitivity, and aid metabolism. These medications mimic GLP-1, a gut hormone released after eating, signaling satiety to your brain and helping you eat less without constant willpower. Additionally, they slow stomach emptying and improve insulin release, reducing blood sugar spikes that often lead to energy crashes or increased cravings. For those who struggle with late-night snacking or frequent hunger shortly after meals, GLP-1's satiety effect can be genuinely trans-formative.

As we know, starting a peptide protocol requires patience and attention. Semaglutide typically begins at 0.25mg once weekly, allowing your body to adjust. This subcutaneous injection is usually administered in the belly or thigh. After four weeks, if side effects are minimal, you may increase to 0.5mg weekly. Liraglutide is different, taken daily starting at a low dose and slowly ramped up over two weeks. For best results, take these medications at consistent times. In the first week or two, you may feel less hungry or slightly queasy after meals, but these symptoms usually lessen as you adjust.

Monitoring your response is as important as the injections. Many women find food relationships change significantly within two weeks, as unplanned snacking may disappear, and smaller portions or skipping dessert may feel natural. Still, some report feeling lightheaded if they skip meals, especially early on. Keeping a craving log can help identify patterns and tweak meal timing and choices for improved stability.

You should also note that gastrointestinal side effects like nausea, bloating, constipation, or mild diarrhea are common with GLP-1 agonists. Manage these by eating smaller, more frequent meals and opting for gentle foods like bananas, rice, or plain chicken if your stomach is upset. Eat slowly and chew thoroughly. Drink water steadily, but not in large amounts at once. If constipation arises, gradually add fiber such as oatmeal or chia seeds.

Weight stalls can still occur. If your weight doesn't change for more than two weeks, and diet or activity haven't shifted, review your protocol. Are you missing doses or eating more treats because hunger is lower? Sometimes stalls reflect metabolic changes, not just plateaus. Re-examine your craving log for subtle changes. If nothing is obvious and you feel well, maintain your dose for a few more weeks before adjusting.

You should pause or cycle off if GI side effects persist after four weeks at the lowest dose, or if fasting blood sugar rises or fatigue continues despite good sleep and nutrition. As always, touch base with your health provider before making changes or if you feel uncertain about your body's reactions.

Sometimes reducing the dose or changing timing helps, but occasionally cycling off is necessary. You can use this template before and during your protocol to help reveal real patterns in hunger and satisfaction.

Troubleshooting Plateaus

Hitting a wall with your progress can be frustrating, especially when you've done everything "right."

You step on the scale, expecting a drop, only to see the same number for days or weeks. But before panic sets in, remember: not every stall is a true plateau. Our bodies are fluid—literally. Hormones, salt intake, sleep, and stress all play tricks with water retention and scale weight, masking fat loss even when changes are happening under the surface. I always tell my clients to zoom out and look at trends over three weeks, not just three days. Pull up your progress log, check your body measurements, and review your photos. Maybe your waist shrank but your weight held steady, or your jeans fit better even though the scale didn't budge. These are signs of normal fluctuations, not failure.

A real plateau usually sticks around for three weeks or more, with zero change in weight, measurements, or body fat despite consistent effort. This is where a troubleshooting mindset matters. I like to break it down with a simple "if-then" flow: If you pause and see the stall is only a week long, chalk it up to water or hormones, especially around your period or after a salty meal. If the stall lingers for three weeks, then it's time to tweak something. Start by **examining your nutrition**: have extra snacks crept in or portions gotten bigger as hunger fades? Sometimes appetite drops so much on peptides that protein slips too low and metabolism slows in response. Boost protein intake for a week and see how your body reacts. Next, **check your activity**: have workouts gotten shorter or less intense? Adding back just one day of strength training or brisk walks can make a big difference.

If diet and movement are on point, you can now examine your

peptide routine. Maybe you started with three doses of Ipamorelin weekly and results were strong at first, but now things have stalled. It might be time to increase to five weekly doses, always watching for side effects or sleep changes. Alternatively, try stacking another peptide like MOTS-c for two weeks to jumpstart fat burning at the cellular level. If you've been on the same protocol for eight weeks straight, consider cycling off for two weeks; sometimes receptors need a chance to reset before responding again.

A practical decision tree looks like this:

Plateau less than two weeks?
Wait it out and monitor stress and sleep.

Plateau for three weeks?

1. *Audit food*: Track honestly for seven days.
2. *Adjust workouts*: Add one session or change intensity.
3. *Review peptide dose*: Consider increasing frequency or adding a new stack if safety allows.
4. Still stuck? *Take a two-week "reset"* break from peptides, focus on sleep and recovery, then restart protocol.

You should also be aware that beyond physical tweaks, there's a psychological side to plateaus that rarely gets enough attention. For one thing, motivation can nosedive when progress slows, triggering self-doubt and frustration. I tell my clients to treat these periods as information-gathering missions instead of failures. Reframe plateaus as signs that your body is consolidating changes or preparing for a "whoosh"—that sudden drop after weeks of nothing happening on the scale. The *whoosh* effect is real: sometimes fat cells hold onto water after shrinking and release it all at once, leading to dramatic changes overnight.

Support is everything during this rollercoaster ride, so get yourself an accountability partner. It could be a friend, a coach, or even an online group that gets the ups and downs of peptide protocols. They're the ones who'll remind you of the non-scale victories: better sleep, clearer skin, a mood boost, or maybe even a new personal best at the gym. Aim for a weekly check-in, even if it's just sharing a sweaty selfie or celebrating the fact that you survived a tough week without throwing in the towel. Because motivation doesn't just come from pure grit; it thrives when we feel seen and cheered on through the setbacks.

And hey, if you catch yourself in a spiral of negative self-talk ("I'm failing," "This will never work"), hit pause. Time for a quick **mindset reset**. What would you say to a friend in your shoes? Probably something a lot kinder than the internal monologue you've got going on. Take a moment to jot down three things that are going well (outside of that pesky scale). Maybe you nailed a stressful day without reaching for junk food, or perhaps you noticed you're less wiped out after work. These small wins? They're like little high-fives from your future self, signaling the kind of change that's happening just under the surface.

Above all, **stay patient and flexible**. Fat loss is rarely linear, especially for women navigating hormonal cycles and life stressors. Just keep showing up, adjusting thoughtfully based on real data (not knee-jerk reactions) and giving yourself credit for every step forward.

Safety First: Monitoring Bloodwork and Minimizing Metabolic Risks

When you start any peptide protocol, especially the ones focused on fat loss or metabolism, safety needs to be your top priority.

It's tempting to just jump in and watch the results, but your body deserves a thoughtful approach. This means checking your baseline health with bloodwork before you even begin, and then tracking how your body responds as you move through your cycle. Knowing your numbers will give you peace of mind and allow you to catch little issues before they turn into big problems.

I always recommend beginning with a set of core labs, which are your health "dashboard." You'll want to check fasting glucose (how your body handles sugar after an overnight fast), HbA1c (shows your average blood sugar trends over a few months), IGF-1 (reflects how much growth hormone activity is happening), liver enzymes (ALT, AST, which flag liver stress), and a lipid panel (cholesterol and triglycerides). Know that these tests aren't just for people with existing health problems; they matter for everyone considering peptide support because they reveal how well your metabolism, liver, and hormones are actually functioning. Even if you feel fine, subtle changes on these labs can point to risk before you notice symptoms.

Interpreting these labs won't require you to memorize every number, but will enable you to recognize what's "off." Let's say your fasting glucose is creeping over 100 mg/dL or your HbA1c starts climbing above 5.7%, that's a cue your body is struggling with sugar. If IGF-1 jumps way beyond the normal range for your age, it could mean you're getting too much growth hormone stimulation from peptides. If ALT or AST (your liver enzymes) rise above normal, your liver may be feeling overloaded. This is especially important since women sometimes metabolize peptides differently than men. And if your LDL cholesterol heads up or triglycerides spike, it's time to review your diet and peptide plan. These red flags signal it's time to pause, reflect, and maybe make changes before things get risky.

Setting up a **monitoring schedule** is straightforward and takes the guesswork out of the process. I tell my clients to **get baseline labs** a week or two before starting any new protocol. This helps spot issues and sets a reference for comparison later.

Four weeks into the protocol, repeat the same labs; this is usually enough time for any major changes to show up. At eight weeks, test again, especially if you're stacking multiple peptides or running consecutive cycles. After finishing a cycle, give yourself two to four weeks off, then repeat labs once more to see how your body recovers. This rhythm lets you catch any issues early and gives you confidence that you're not missing silent side effects.

Now, what do you do if the numbers aren't perfect? If fasting glucose or HbA1c jumps higher than where you started, or if liver enzymes move out of range, stop the peptides and check in with your healthcare provider before continuing. The same goes for symptoms: If you notice persistent nausea, jaundice (yellowing skin or eyes), severe fatigue, swelling in your limbs, or dark urine, pause everything and seek medical advice. These are not moments to power through; they're signals to take seriously. Sometimes it's as simple as adjusting the dose or taking a longer break between cycles. Other times, you may need a different protocol altogether.

Keep up with **healthy habits**: stay hydrated, eat lots of fiber and colorful veggies, move daily, and make quality rest and sleep non-negotiable. These basics help buffer any metabolic stress from peptides and keep your results sustainable.

Checklist: When to "Pause & Call"

- Fasting glucose >110 mg/dL
- HbA1c above 5.7%
- IGF-1 outside normal range for age/gender
- ALT or AST above upper limit of normal
- New or worsening fatigue that doesn't resolve with rest
- Yellowing of skin/eyes or dark urine
- Swelling in hands/feet

- Persistent nausea or loss of appetite

Smart peptide biohacking revolves around teaming up with your body. The best results come when you're patient, so take the time to listen to what your body is telling you now. Trust me, the rewards are so much sweeter when you don't rush the process.

FIVE

PEPTIDE BIOHACKS FOR HORMONE BALANCE, MOOD, AND COGNITIVE UPGRADE

Hormones can sometimes make you feel out of control, snapping over little things, being emotional for no reason, or struggling with night sweats and sleeplessness. It's frustrating when your body feels unpredictable and the usual advice is just to accept it. Instead, peptides offer a targeted approach to regaining some balance in these challenging times, not as miracle cures, but as tools that help support your body's natural rhythms.

Some peptides specifically regulate reproductive hormones, energy, metabolism, and sleep. For women, two noteworthy peptides are KISS-1 and CJC-1295. KISS-1 (mimicking "kisspeptin") helps regulate reproductive hormone cycles and signaling. If you have irregular cycles, intense PMS, or erratic mood swings, KISS-1 can encourage your brain to naturally balance hormones like LH and FSH, helpful in both unpredictable periods and perimenopause.

CJC-1295 takes a different approach by signaling your pituitary gland to increase natural growth hormone release. During perimenopause and menopause, declining growth hormone leads to fatigue, disrupted sleep, increased abdominal fat, and more hormone-related symptoms. CJC-1295 helps gently restore growth hormone levels, which can lead to better sleep, improved mood, and a sense of vitality, especially as estrogen wanes. It doesn't replace hormones, but rather supports the hormonal system.

Wondering if peptides could help? Consider: Are your cycles irregular or skipped? Is your PMS overwhelming with mood swings, tenderness, pain? Are hot flashes or night sweats ruining your sleep? Has menopause left you foggy or irritable? If yes, you might benefit from exploring peptide protocols focused on hormonal balance.

Matching symptoms to peptides will allow you to personalize your approach. For PMS relief (especially severe moodiness, cravings, or cramps) KISS-1 can be used in the luteal phase, which is after ovulation, before your period. Typical use involves every-other-day subcutaneous injections for 10–12 days before your period. Most women notice reduced irritability, cravings, and cramps within a cycle or two. While it's not instant, significant improvement is frequently seen by the second month.

For perimenopausal insomnia, anxiety, or mood swings, CJC-1295 combined with lifestyle changes (mindfulness, movement) can be effective. This peptide is usually injected 2–3 times per week at bedtime, starting with a low dose (100–200 mcg) and adjusting as tolerated. Noticeable effects (deeper sleep, steadier moods, subtle body composition shifts) often appear after 4–6 weeks.

If you use hormone replacement therapy (HRT), bioidentical hormones, or supplements (like chasteberry or magnesium), peptides typically can be integrated safely, but always involve your hormone provider. Peptides may complement HRT by supporting underlying regulatory pathways without adding synthetic hormones. Coordination is essential: discuss planned protocols with your provider, never stop prescribed medications without supervision, and avoid doubling up on estrogenic agents unless guided by a professional.

For best results, pair peptides with healthy lifestyle shifts. Again, track your symptoms daily: record mood, cramps, sleep, hot flashes, etc. Eat an anti-inflammatory diet and opt for gentle movement on tough days (like yoga or walking). Magnesium glycinate may reduce cramps and improve sleep, but always clear new supplements or protocols with your doctor if you're on medication.

Hormone Harmony Checklist

- Irregular or skipped cycles?
- Severe PMS (mood swings, bloating, pain)?
- Perimenopausal or menopausal symptoms (hot flashes, insomnia, mood changes)?
- Tried lifestyle changes without relief?
- Willing to track symptoms and communicate with your provider?

If you check at least two, peptide-based protocols could be worth discussing with your gynecologist.

Everyone deserves stability and relief from hormonal chaos. But, as always, safety first: Begin with low doses and increase slowly. Peptides such as KISS-1 and CJC-1295 are generally very well-tolerated when sourced from legitimate providers and used with supervision. Minor side effects may include slight injection site redness or mild headache. When adding peptides to other regimens, make changes gradually (two weeks apart) to track effects clearly.

Mood-Boosting Peptides

If you ever feel stuck in a stress spiral (on edge, your mind racing, or easily pushed over the edge), know that this isn't just being "too sensitive." Women's brains and bodies often respond intensely to stress and mood triggers, sometimes more than you'd like. This is where mood-supporting peptides, such as Selank and Semax, can support your nervous system and stress resilience, offering stability during overwhelming times.

Selank gently boosts the GABA system, the brain's primary calming network. GABA (gamma-aminobutyric acid) acts as a natural anti-anxiety brake. As a nasal spray, Selank increases GABA activity, helping you feel less anxious and more grounded, even during chaos. It can also lower cortisol, reducing that "wired-but-tired" feeling common during busy or emotional weeks when you hardly catch your breath. If you're stressed before deadlines, or PMS brings irritability and worry, Selank may bring noticeable calm, especially if stress manifests physically with jaw tension, headaches, or sleep issues.

Semax works differently, boosting neurotrophic factors like BDNF (brain-derived neurotrophic factor), to support healthy brain cells, learning, memory, and emotional stability. Instead of just muting anxiety, it helps your brain recover from stress. Semax is helpful for mood dips in your cycle's second half, postpartum lows, or menopause blues. It's also favored by women juggling high-stress work and family life, since it clears your mind without causing jitteriness or an energy crash.

Timing your use makes a difference. Selank is best for acute stress, such as upcoming demanding work weeks or emotional challenges. Use Selank nasal spray two to three times daily. Typical dosing is 250–400 mcg per spray for five to seven days, pausing afterward. During PMS, Selank can smooth emotional swings and calm racing thoughts. For anxious or overstimulated postpartum moms wanting to avoid sedating medications, Selank is a gentle option.

Semax suits longer-term mood dips, such as the luteal phase, chronic work stress, or post-menopause changes. Usual doses are 300–600 mcg per nostril once or twice daily, for up to 14 days. Many women notice lighter moods and sharper thinking within three to five days. If both peptides seem necessary during a tough month, alternate them to avoid overwhelming your system.

Track your progress with a mood tracking app (Daylio, Mood-notes) or by jotting daily notes on your phone or journal. Rate your mood each day (1–10), and track anxiety, energy, irritability, or sleep. After two to three weeks, see if you're less anxious, recovering from stress faster, mentally clearer, and less tearful. These shifts usually indicate the peptides are working. If you notice little or no change after 21 days (even after adjusting dose or timing) you might not respond to that specific peptide.

Also, be aware of interactions. If you take antidepressants (SSRIs like fluoxetine or sertraline), benzodiazepines (like alprazolam), or herbal adaptogens (ashwagandha, rhodiola), consult your doctor before starting peptides. Selank and Semax rarely cause issues, but using them with sedatives or anti-anxiety meds can result in drowsiness or stronger effects. Adaptogens may also change how peptides are processed, so add new supplements one at a time.

Make sure to check your medications for SSRIs, SNRIs, benzodiazepines, sleep meds (zolpidem), antihistamines, or mood stabilizers before starting. For your doctor, you can mention: "I'm interested in trying Selank/Semax for stress and mood support. I currently take [list all meds]. Are there any concerns about interactions? Should I adjust timing or dosage?" This shows your proactive approach and helps them guide you properly.

Mood-Tracking Self-Check

- Am I recovering faster from stress?
- Do tense moments feel calmer?
- Is sleep deeper or more restful?
- Are anxious thoughts or irritability down?
- Do I feel clearer or more motivated?

If you answer yes to most after two weeks, and have no major side effects, your approach is on track. If not, discuss protocol changes with your doctor or consider other options.

Cognitive Enhancement

Have you ever experienced cognitive fog, forgetting why you entered a room or struggling to focus at your computer? With work, family, constant notifications, and shifting hormones, our brains sometimes need extra support. Peptides like GHK-Cu and nootropics such as Noopept offer practical ways to enhance memory, focus, and creativity when you need a mental boost.

GHK-Cu might not be mainstream, but it's effective. This copper peptide works at the cellular level, stimulating brain-derived neurotrophic factor (BDNF)—essentially "brain fertilizer"—to promote synaptic plasticity, the brain's ability to adapt, rewire, and store information. GHK-Cu supports long-term brain health and learning, providing benefits that go beyond a brief boost. Nasal spray delivery is popular for its direct effect without injections or pills. Many users, especially busy professionals and multitasking moms, report improved idea flow and less distraction when using GHK-Cu before creative work or periods requiring deep focus.

Noopept brings another angle. This synthetic peptide-like compound increases acetylcholine, a neurotransmitter critical for attention, reasoning, and quick learning. With higher acetylcholine, thoughts connect more smoothly, making mental processing quicker and sharper. Noopept not only increases alertness; it can contribute to long-term brain health through mild neuroprotective effects. It's usually taken orally as a tablet under the tongue or with water, about 30–60 minutes before needing to perform at your mental best. For exam prep, high-stakes meetings, or demanding days, Noopept boosts focus without caffeine's jitters.

Protocols for these enhancers are simple and most effective when used consistently. For GHK-Cu, start with one spray (50–100 mcg) per nostril in the morning, repeating in the afternoon if needed, up to five times per week. Noopept dosage begins at 10–20 mg once daily, not to exceed two doses a day, and is best taken earlier to avoid insomnia. Consider using GHK-Cu before creative work in the morning and Noopept in the afternoon for pure focus.

When it comes to cognitive enhancers, safety should always be front and center. GHK-Cu and Noopept are usually kind to the brain when taken at the right doses, but overdoing it can bring on headaches, irritability, and—unfortunately—more brain fog. A headache is often your brain's way of saying, "Hey, slow down, I'm not a machine!" So, take a breather or dial back your dose if that happens. If you find yourself overstimulated or having trouble winding down, it's probably time to hit pause on your regimen for a bit. Keep it in check by sticking to cycles of four to eight weeks, followed by at least two weeks off. Your brain will thank you, and so will your tolerance levels.

Want to supercharge your results? Make sure your habits are as brain-friendly as your supplements. Meditation isn't just for the zen masters or those weirdly calm people at yoga class. A quick, mindful breathing session before you take GHK-Cu or Noopept can prep your brain for laser focus. And those blue light-blocking glasses? Not just for looking cool (though they do that too). They help protect your sleep cycle so your brain can actually rest. Stay hydrated and make sure your meals include brain-boosting goodies like eggs, which are full of choline to keep those neurotransmitters firing on all cylinders.

Now, here's the secret sauce: track your progress. I know this keeps coming up, and it's not about obsessing, but about knowing if these brain-boosters are actually doing their job. Once a week, check in with yourself: Can you recall yesterday's details? Are you powering through tasks like a productivity machine? And how's your mental flexibility? Can you juggle tasks without feeling like you're drowning in a sea of to-do lists? Use a simple app or checklist to make this painless. And here's a little productivity hack: pick a time each day and pair your peptide or nootropic dose with a focused work block. Turn off those pesky notifications, and give yourself 40 minutes of undistracted time to crush your top priority.

Weekly Cognitive Self-Assessment

- ☑ How easily do I recall names and tasks?
- ☑ Can I switch between projects without losing my train of thought?
- ☑ Are my ideas clearer or more creative than last week?
- ☑ Do I recover quickly from distractions?
- ☑ Any headaches or new symptoms?

If things start going south (like, headaches that won't quit or focus that's as elusive as a unicorn) go back to the basics. Check your hydration, your rest, and any new lifestyle changes. And yes, don't forget to take breaks from the supplements. If things still aren't right, don't hesitate to call in a health professional. Sometimes it's stress or a sneaky nutrient deficiency causing the hiccup. Use these reflection questions as your weekly "cognitive dashboard."

Hormonal Fluctuations: Adapting Protocols for Your Cycle

. Tuning your peptide routine to your body's natural rhythm can make all the difference. If you've ever tried a supplement that worked wonders one month, then fizzled the next, you're not imagining things. Your menstrual cycle is a moving target, shifting hormone levels every few days, and that means your body's response to peptides can change just as quickly.

The two main phases—follicular (from your period to ovulation) and luteal (after ovulation until your next bleed)—each bring their own mix of energy, cravings, mood, and even how well peptides work for you. During the follicular phase, estrogen rises, and most women feel more clear-headed, energetic, and socially bold. Peptide dosing often feels smoother here; your body tends to recover quicker and tolerate higher doses without side effects. You might notice sharper focus or better workouts when using cognitive or metabolic peptides in this window. As you slip into the luteal phase, progesterone takes over. This hormone can slow you down, making you more sensitive to stress and sometimes less tolerant of certain stacks. Some women find they need to lower their peptide dose to avoid headaches or bloating, while others benefit from shifting timing, moving an evening dose earlier to support sleep or swapping in peptides that soothe rather than stimulate.

Navigating perimenopause or menopause adds another layer of unpredictability. You might go weeks without a period, or your symptoms may shift from month to month. Estrogen levels can swing from high to low overnight, making your response to peptides less consistent. You may find that a stack that worked last season now leaves you jittery or sleepless. When estrogen drops, your body often becomes more sensitive to change. This is when ongoing self-monitoring pays off. If you notice more hot flashes, anxiety, or trouble sleeping after starting or increasing a peptide, back down on the dose or give yourself longer breaks between cycles. Listen for subtle clues: are you waking up at 3 a.m.? Is your mood less stable than usual? Adjusting protocols as estrogen declines might mean reducing stimulating stacks, focusing on gentler support, or adding longer rest periods between cycles.

Whether you're tracking regular periods or dealing with unpredictable cycles, keep another log to help you spot patterns and adapt your peptide use in real time. No need for fancy apps, a simple chart works wonders.

Try this template: each row is a day of your cycle; columns include "Period/Spotting," "Mood," "Energy," "Cognitive Clarity," and "Peptide Dose." Jot down symptoms and dosing changes each day so you can see at a glance how hormones and peptides are playing together. For instance, if you notice migraines mid-cycle whenever you increase a peptide dose, try lowering the amount or splitting it across morning and night. If breakthrough bleeding pops up when stacking peptides during ovulation, pause the protocol until bleeding stops and restart with a lower dose the next cycle.

Troubleshooting can feel like detective work at times. If you hit an unexpected wall (no improvements, new side effects, or plateaus) consider where you are in your cycle first. Sometimes a protocol needs a simple tweak: lower the dose during PMS if moodiness spikes, shift timing if sleep is off, or pause for a full cycle if you experience breakthrough bleeding or migraines that don't resolve quickly. For women prone to mid-cycle headaches or energy crashes, holding off on stimulating peptides until after ovulation often helps. If fatigue or irritability shows up in the luteal phase despite protocol adjustments, switch focus to peptides that support relaxation and sleep instead of those designed for high energy.

For those dealing with long gaps between periods or unpredictable perimenopausal symptoms, give yourself permission to experiment with longer rest phases. Sometimes, two weeks on, two weeks off feels better than rigid monthly cycles. If you notice certain symptoms always track with specific peptides or timing, then you'll know to adjust accordingly for the next round.

Cycle Tracking Template
(Peptide Protocol + Period Log)

Day	Period/Spotting	Mood	Energy	Cognitive Clarity	Peptide Dose
Day 1	Period/Spotting	3/10	5/10	10/10	None
Day 7	Period/Spotting	8/10	8/10	10/10	1 spray AM
Day 14	Ovulation	8/10	9/10	10/10	1 spray AM
Day 21	PMS	5/10	6/10	10/10	½ dose PM
Day 28	Spotting	3/10	4/10	10/10	Paused

This kind of log will help you become your own expert and give your provider real information if things get complicated. Plus, staying flexible and honest with yourself will help turn monthly hormone chaos into an opportunity for real progress, rather than just survival.

Managing Interactions: Peptides, Medications, and Safety Checklists

Navigating the world of peptides is empowering, but it's never just about what you add to your routine; it's also about protecting yourself from unwanted surprises.

Mixing peptides with medications, supplements, or therapies you already use deserves careful thought. The key is to stay proactive and informed, not anxious. Many women have prescriptions for antidepressants, thyroid meds, hormone therapies, or sleep aids. Layer on a peptide protocol, and the question becomes: "Will this cocktail play nice, or will it create chaos?" You don't have to guess. Building a framework for safe combinations means knowing what to look for, what to avoid, and when to throw up the red flag.

Let's start with common interaction points. If you use SSRIs (like sertraline or fluoxetine), sleep medications (zolpidem, melatonin), or hormone therapies (oral contraceptives, bioidentical estrogen), always check for known conflicts. For instance, some peptides can intensify the effects of sleep meds, leading to excessive grogginess or even confusion in some women. SSRIs and peptides rarely interact at a chemical level, but mood swings or agitation that pop up suddenly mean it's time to pause and reassess, especially if mood destabilization is new for you.

Hormone therapy combined with peptides often works well, but if you notice increased breast tenderness, headaches, or unexpected bleeding, step back and consult both your peptide-savvy provider and your gynecologist.

Here's a quick reference chart you can keep handy:

Medication Type	Possible Interaction	What to Watch For
SSRIs (sertraline etc.)	Rare; occasional mood changes	Agitation, sadness, sleep issues
Sleep meds (zolpidem)	Possible additive sedation	Grogginess, confusion
Hormone therapy (HRT)	Mild overlap; possible increased sensitivity	Headaches, breast tenderness
Stimulants (ADHD meds)	Rare; possible anxiety or racing thoughts	Jitters, insomnia
Thyroid meds	No direct interaction expected	Overcalm or overstimulated states

Now, no one wants to think about things going wrong. But knowing red flag symptoms helps you act fast and safely.

Severe headaches that come on suddenly and don't respond to hydration or rest should never be ignored; stop the protocol and reach out to your doctor immediately.

Allergic reactions sometimes show up as hives, swelling of lips or tongue, or trouble breathing; this is an emergency, call 911 or get help without delay.

Mood destabilization goes beyond a rough day; if you experience sudden sadness, anxiety that keeps you from functioning, or thoughts that scare you, stop your protocol and contact a mental health professional right away.

Other stop-now scenarios include chest pain, fainting, unexplained swelling in the legs, or new neurological symptoms.

I always encourage women to keep a safety checklist on hand for every protocol. For each peptide routine (whether it's for mood, focus, or hormone balance) write down: the name of the peptide; your starting dose; current medications/supplements; the date you started; expected benefits (so you know what "normal" looks like); possible side effects; and your doctor's contact info.

Every time you make a change (increase a dose, add a supplement, swap out medications) note the date and reason in your log. For doctor appointments, arrive prepared. Bring your symptom log and protocol list. Include dates and doses, and note any side effects or new symptoms with their timelines. In case of emergency (sudden swelling, breathing trouble), stop all new protocols and seek care immediately. Do not wait it out.

Safety Monitoring Checklist

- List all current medications and supplements
- Note start/end dates of each peptide protocol
- Record daily symptoms: mood/energy/cognition/physical changes
- Check weekly for trends or side effects
- Flag any red flag symptoms for immediate medical review
- Bring updated logs to every doctor appointment

Alright, ladies, let's wrap this up with the most important thing you need to remember: safety is all about the details. Keep track of what you're taking and how you're feeling, so nothing slips through the cracks.

Peptides? They absolutely have a place in your complex routines, but only if you're paying attention to the little things.

SIX

PEPTIDE BIOHACKS FOR SKIN, HAIR, AND BEAUTY

We've all been there, standing in front of the mirror, staring at those new lines or stubborn spots that seem to have appeared overnight, despite our best efforts with every cream promising miracle results. It's frustrating, to say the least. Sometimes we wish for something more than just the usual surface treatments. Something that works from the inside out. Enter peptides, the skincare superheroes.

First up: GHK-Cu. Sounds like a fancy name, right? Well, it's a peptide that's naturally found in your plasma (though, like all good things, it tends to decline as we age). This little powerhouse is a cellular signal that tells your fibroblasts to get busy making collagen and elastin, which are essentially the building blocks of firm, bouncy skin. Think of it like sending a memo to your skin to "Get your act together, stat!" But it's not just about firmness. GHK-Cu also reduces inflammation, fights free radicals, and helps speed up recovery from post-acne marks or sensitivity. Basically, it's the Swiss army knife of skin repair. Clinical studies back it up, showing that it can thicken skin, improve elasticity, and even fade those pesky dark spots. If you've noticed that your wounds take longer to heal or your skin is feeling a little thinner, this peptide could be your new best friend.

Now, onto Melanotan II. This one works a little differently. It mimics your body's natural melanocyte-stimulating hormone (yes, that's a real thing, not just something out of a sci-fi movie). What does that mean for you? Well, it boosts melanin production—aka, your skin's natural tanning pigment—without the need for sun exposure. It's a game-changer if you burn easily or prefer to skip the sun damage altogether. Plus, it can help smooth out uneven skin tone, hide scars, or even make those veins a little less noticeable. But proceed with caution: get the dosage wrong, and you might end up with dark spots, new moles, or blotchy skin. So, like with all good things, moderation is key.

When it comes to using these peptides, how you apply them really matters. With GHK-Cu, start slow. A couple of drops of a topical serum after cleansing, on damp skin, before you slather on your moisturizer or sunscreen. If you're using actives like vitamin C or retinoids, apply GHK-Cu first. It absorbs fast and won't mess with your makeup. Sensitive skin? Try it every other night to start, then increase to nightly use if all goes well. For deep scars or wrinkles, massage in a couple of extra drops. Feeling extra adventurous? Microinjections (under medical guidance, of course) can do wonders for stubborn areas, but don't jump into that without a professional's approval.

Melanotan II is a little more hands-on. To get that subtle glow, start with a small dose, around 100 mcg under the skin every other day for the first week. Slowly increase it as you start to see some color. Don't go overboard, more is not better here. Stick to the recommended doses, or you could end up with uneven coloring, especially if you've got freckles or moles. A typical "tanning" cycle lasts 2 to 4 weeks, followed by a nice, long break. Don't rush the process; your skin will thank you.

Remember, not every peptide is for everyone. If you've got fine lines, slower healing skin, or past scarring, GHK-Cu could be your new go-to. It's especially great if you have fair or sensitive skin (hello, rosacea), since it's soothing and anti-inflammatory. Melanotan II is best for those with fair skin who burn easily and struggle to tan. If you've got a history of melanoma or skin pigment issues like vitiligo, though, skip it. There are plenty of other options out there that'll suit your needs.

Quick Screening Checklist

- Fitzpatrick skin type? (Types I–III gain the most from Melanotan II.)
- Time spent in direct sun? (If high, be cautious with Melanotan II to avoid extra pigment.)
- Allergic reactions to copper or topical peptides? (Do a patch test before full application.)
- Sensitive/reactive skin? (Start GHK-Cu slowly, watching for redness or itching.)

As always, safety comes first. For GHK-Cu serums, always patch test behind the ear, and wait 24 hours for any redness before applying to your face. Don't use over fresh wounds or broken skin. With injections, use only sterile equipment and rotate sites to avoid lumps or irritation. Melanotan II users should regularly check skin for new spots, changes in freckles, or darkening areas and stop immediately if anything seems amiss, then see a dermatologist. Side effects could include nausea, flushing, appetite changes, or mood shifts at higher doses.

Peptide Insights

In natural light, examine your skin without makeup or filters. What do you want to see change by next season (e.g., brighter tone, smoother scars, reduced redness)? Write down three goals as your "before" reference as you explore peptides.

_____

_____

_____

_____

_____

_____

_____

_____

_____

_____

Hair Growth and Restoration

Hair loss can chip away at your confidence in a way few other health changes do. The brush full of strands, the widening part, the feeling of your scalp peeking through; these moments are personal and often emotional. For women, hair thinning isn't just about looks. It's tangled up with identity, stress, hormones, and even life events like childbirth or menopause. So it's no wonder many women are searching for answers beyond the typical drugstore aisle.

Thymosin Beta-4 (TB-4) is one of the most promising peptides for hair restoration. What sets TB-4 apart is its ability to trigger angiogenesis. Basically, it helps your body build new micro-blood vessels around sluggish follicles. This means more nutrients and oxygen reach the roots, gently nudging dormant hairs back into growth mode. TB-4 also wakes up stem cells in the hair bulge region, which is where new growth starts. For women with thinning all over (not just a receding hairline), this is a game changer. TB-4 calms inflammation on the scalp, too, which is crucial if you're dealing with sensitivity or redness after styling, coloring, or stress.

GHK-Cu isn't just for skin, it's a star for scalp health as well. This copper peptide can lower inflammation that chokes off follicles and helps boost the number of active hair-producing cells. GHK-Cu signals your body to ramp up collagen and glycosaminoglycan production in the scalp, making each strand look denser and feel stronger. It's particularly helpful if your hair feels brittle or you've noticed more fallout than usual in the shower.

You don't have to guess where to start. For at-home support, you can mix your own GHK-Cu scalp serum: dilute 2 mg of GHK-Cu peptide in 20 mL of sterile saline or distilled water, then add a few drops of a gentle carrier like aloe vera gel for staying power. Apply 1–2 mL to your scalp nightly, focusing on sparse areas. Massage in gently and let dry before bed; no need to rinse out. For even better absorption, pair this with a microneedling routine once a week. Use a dermaroller with 0.5 mm needles (never share or reuse) on clean, dry scalp before applying the peptide serum. Short, gentle passes are enough; don't press hard or cause bleeding. Aftercare is simple: avoid harsh shampoos and give your scalp 24 hours to recover before styling or washing.

TB-4 is available as a topical or, more effectively, as a subcutaneous injection (usually 2–5 mg twice weekly for 6–8 weeks under professional guidance). Some clinics also combine TB-4 with PRP or other growth factors for stubborn cases. If you're postpartum or experiencing hormone-driven shedding (like telogen effluvium), consider starting with gentle topical GHK-Cu first. It's safe for most nursing moms and doesn't disrupt your hormones further. If you're noticing rapid shedding after giving birth, don't panic. This is often temporary and linked to hormonal swings rather than permanent follicle loss.

Women's hair loss is rarely as straightforward as it is for men. Female pattern hair loss often shows up as diffuse thinning over the crown rather than receding temples, so tracking changes can be subtle at first. Postpartum shedding hits fast and hard, usually 2–4 months after delivery, while perimenopausal thinning might sneak up over years. For hormonal cases, it helps to use peptides alongside lifestyle tweaks: stress reduction, scalp massage, and a balanced diet rich in iron and protein.

Sticking with a routine makes a big difference. Some women experience an initial "shedding phase" when peptides kick-start the hair cycle, so don't freak out if you see more hairs at first; this often means old hairs are dropping so new ones can push through. Keep a log of how often you apply serums or do microneedling sessions, and note any irritation, redness, or sensitivity. If your scalp feels sore or you develop flakiness, cut back frequency to every other night or switch to a lower concentration while your skin adapts.

If you feel stuck or see no change after three months, reassess: Are you consistent? Is there an underlying thyroid issue or nutrient gap holding you back? Sometimes it takes tweaking your protocol, maybe spacing out microneedling more if your scalp is sensitive, or layering in nutrition support (like biotin or omega-3s) for stubborn cases. If you hit a wall, check with a dermatologist who understands peptides and women's hair loss.

Reducing Wrinkles and Hyperpigmentation

If you've ever caught your reflection in bright morning light and noticed new lines or the uneven shadow of a sunspot, you know how personal skin care can feel. We want real changes: less creasing around the eyes, softer smile lines, and a more even glow. For tackling wrinkles and patches of hyperpigmentation, I've seen the best results come from stepwise, layered protocols that blend peptides with classic skincare staples and a bit of patience.

Phase 1 starts with foundation: collagen-boosting peptides and hydration. Collagen is what keeps skin plump, bouncy, and less prone to lines, but its production drops steadily after our twenties. Begin with a simple evening routine. After cleansing, pat your face dry and apply a hydrating toner or mist such as rosewater or a light hyaluronic acid spray. While your skin is still damp, press in a serum containing collagen-supporting peptides. These serums work best when layered under richer creams; let the peptide soak in for a minute, then follow with your favorite moisturizer to lock in moisture. This step is non-negotiable for anyone fighting dehydration lines or feeling that tight, papery sensation after washing.

In the same evening, layer on a low-strength retinol (0.25–0.5%). Retinol accelerates cell turnover, encouraging fresher skin to emerge and helping peptides reach deeper layers. If you're new to retinol or have sensitive skin, start with twice weekly applications and increase slowly as tolerated. You'll want to buffer retinol with your moisturizer at first to lower the risk of dryness or flaking. If you're already comfortable with retinoids, alternate nights between peptides and retinol to avoid irritation.

For your mornings, vitamin C takes the stage. It's a potent antioxidant and supports collagen synthesis while brightening pigment irregularities. Use a few drops of vitamin C serum on clean skin, then layer your daytime peptide serum if you like. Always finish with broad-spectrum sunscreen (SPF 30 or higher) since unprotected sun exposure will undo all your hard work, and can actually worsen pigmentation when using actives.

Phase 2 is for stubborn pigment: targeted peptides paired with gentle exfoliation and, for some, microdosed Melanotan II under medical guidance. Start this phase once your skin tolerates the basics without irritation, usually after 4–6 weeks of nightly peptides and retinol. Every other night, use a mild exfoliant (like lactic acid or mandelic acid pads) before your peptide serum to boost penetration. For women with darker skin tones or anyone prone to post-inflammatory hyperpigmentation (PIH), opt for mandelic acid or polyhydroxy acids, as they're less likely to trigger irritation or rebound darkening. Be extra cautious with exfoliants and always patch test new products, since PIH can be stubborn and slow to fade if triggered by over-exfoliation or harsh actives.

Progress with these routines won't be instant, but most women notice smoother texture within four weeks as fine lines begin to soften, and makeup sits better on the skin. By eight weeks, deeper wrinkles start to look less etched in; pigment fades enough that foundation shades may shift lighter or look more even. At twelve weeks of consistent use, you should see noticeable changes in before/after photos: crow's feet flatten, marionette lines soften, and sunspots lose their sharp edges.

At-Home vs. Clinical Use

Deciding between at-home peptide routines and clinical treatments can be daunting, particularly if you're new to both. More women are exploring self-directed beauty solutions, but clinical options are still valuable and empowering. Everyone's situation is unique, so let's clearly compare the essentials: results, cost, convenience, and safety, without glossing over the compromises.

At-home peptide protocols are now highly accessible. A quality GHK-Cu serum or solution can be ordered online, used with simple instructions, and integrated into a daily routine. The benefits are obvious: you control the process, avoid appointment fees, and can adjust your approach at your own pace. Costs range from $35 to $150 per peptide serum (for 4–6 weeks), and an initial setup, including microneedling tools, generally totals $200–$300 for several months of care. These steps fit easily into an existing routine and can be paused or resumed at any time. However, you are responsible for monitoring results, maintaining hygiene, and recognizing early signs of irritation or problems. There is a learning curve: mixing powders, sanitizing tools, and remaining consistent all require vigilance.

In-office procedures such as microneedling or mesotherapy provide greater precision and intensity. Licensed professionals use medical-grade devices that penetrate deeper than home rollers, meaning peptides are delivered more effectively and results may be visible sooner—sometimes after only one session. The cost, however, is significantly higher: $350–$800 per session for microneedling with peptides is typical, and three to six sessions are usually needed for results. Injectable peptide treatments for hair or facial benefits run $150–$400 per area. With this higher cost comes sterile technique, expert protocols, and monitoring of side effects. The advantage here is customized recommendations, troubleshooting by experts, and peace of mind concerning safety.

The best option depends on your lifestyle, comfort with needles or devices, and budget. DIY-ers who like tracking results and are patient with gradual progress often find at-home routines suitable, provided they are diligent about research and safety. For more significant concerns like stubborn wrinkles, pronounced pigment, or serious thinning, or for anyone wanting swift results, clinical treatments can be worth the investment. Professional support is also ideal for those with complicated medical backgrounds, sensitive skin, or issues staying consistent.

To decide, use this approach: If you have mild to moderate issues, start with at-home care for 8–12 weeks. If results are minimal, stall after dedicated use, or if you experience deeper-set lines or significant thinning, it's time to consult a professional. Professional evaluation is especially important if your history includes allergies, autoimmune conditions, or other complexities.

Clinician choice matters greatly. Don't just pick the first med spa you see online; choose providers who disclose their credentials and have demonstrated experience with peptide procedures. Seek board-certified dermatologists or licensed aestheticians skilled in cosmetic injectables and microneedling. Good clinics emphasize infection control with single-use needles, freshly mixed serums, and strict hygiene. Ask whether they use FDA-cleared devices and source peptides from accredited compounding pharmacies. Always read independent reviews and confirm the practitioner has a solid track record with clients similar to you in terms of skin, age, or hair type.

Clinician Choice Checklist

- Is the provider board-certified or licensed?
- Do they explain risks clearly?
- Can they present before/after images of similar cases?
- Is their environment visibly clean with clear safety protocols?
- Are they forthright answering specific technical questions?

If you hear vague assurances of universal results or notice unsafe practices such as reused needles, leave immediately.

Make sure to **advocate for yourself** at every appointment. If you're unsure how to start, try: "I've been researching peptide treatments for my skin/hair. Can you explain what you offer and how safety is maintained?" Follow up with, "What experience do you have treating women of my skin tone/hair type/sensitivity?" Finally, ask, "What side effects should I watch for at home, and how can I contact you with concerns?" Insist on clarification if anything seems unclear or incomplete, and request written protocols when needed.

Your **comfort and safety should always come first.** Whether you prefer at-home routines or professional care, the key is choosing an approach that fits your needs while making informed decisions, not ones based on pressure or trends.

In a Nutshell...

At-Home Peptides: Accessible, budget-friendly, and flexible. Great for those who enjoy self-care, but requires vigilance in research, hygiene, and consistency. Costs range from $35–$300 for setup and supplies.

Clinical Treatments: Professional microneedling and injectable peptide treatments offer faster, more intense results with higher precision. Expect to pay $350–$800 per session, but you get expert care, customized treatments, and peace of mind about safety.

The Best Fit for You: If you're patient and have mild concerns, start at home. Track your progress and, if needed, seek a professional for faster results or serious skin issues.

Choosing a Provider: Be picky. Look for board-certified experts, clean practices, and transparency. Always ask about safety, experience, and results. Trust your instincts and don't settle for vague answers.

Tracking Your Progress

Starting a new skin or hair routine often makes you impatient for results, leading you to question if your efforts are paying off. This is completely normal, which is why a structured system for tracking progress is invaluable.

Small improvements can be hard to spot, and relying on memory isn't reliable. I always suggest beginning a photo journal: take a few minutes every Sunday morning to snap pictures, using natural light in the same spot at a consistent angle. Avoid filters or makeup; you want an honest record of your progress. For faces, photograph from the front, both sides, and close-ups of problem areas. For hair or scalp, try an overhead photo with help, or use a selfie stick to document thinning or regrowth areas. If you're targeting your décolletage (chest/neck), include that zone too, since sun damage and texture changes are common there. Create a straightforward grid in a notes app or on paper to record the date, protocol, lighting details, and quick observations like "less redness" or "new baby hairs." Over weeks, these images and notes give a trustworthy record that a mirror just can't provide.

Photos are important, but objective data offers even more clarity. Try tracking markers like collagen density and skin hydration:

many beauty stores now sell handheld skin analyzers, which estimate hydration and provide an elasticity or "collagen" score. Check the same spot weekly and log your numbers. You'll notice patterns: moisture jumps after you add peptides, or firmness improves with consistency. For hair, scalp health is as important as new strands. Track issues like flakiness, redness, or soreness, as well as whether the scalp feels itchy or tight; these signs may indicate irritation or the need to adjust product frequency. Note any thickening or less visible scalp as a positive trend.

Here's the most important bit: manage your expectations. Instant transformations sound nice in theory, but skin and hair have their own timing, and they're not interested in rushing. Peptide regimens usually take at least four weeks to show small improvements. Full-on changes, like firming or spot-fading, can take up to twelve weeks. Hair regrowth? Well, it's even slower. During the first three weeks, you might notice more shedding as your follicles reset—don't panic, it's temporary. By weeks 4–8, you might spot early signs of new growth. But the real thickening and density you're hoping for? That usually takes anywhere from three to six months. So, be patient, and remember: maintenance is key to holding on to all that progress.

A timeline chart can help keep you motivated and realistic.

For hair:

- Weeks 1–3: temporary shedding
- Weeks 4–12: new growth
- Months 3–6: thickening
- After month 6: maintenance.

For skin:

- Week 4: First hints of glow
- Week 8: Fewer fine lines
- Week 12: Improved firmness.

There will be times when progress stalls or something unexpected happens; maybe photos look unchanged at eight weeks or hair growth plateaus. This is normal—not a failure. Troubleshoot by reviewing your log: have you missed doses, changed products, been very stressed, or switched up your diet? If you've been inconsistent, or layered on too many new items, go back to basics. Sometimes you need to switch up brands or slightly increase product frequency to reignite progress. If irritation, redness, or breakouts occur, pause all actives for five to seven days, then restart gradually with just one product at a time.

Beauty Biohacks

Sometimes, we just want more from our skincare routine than another cream or serum promising miracles. We crave results that feel real, that we can see and touch. That's where combining peptides with beauty tech like red light therapy and microcurrent comes into play. These methods don't replace the basics but elevate them, turning an ordinary regimen into something much more powerful.

Red light therapy, for example, gives your skin cells a burst of energy. It works by activating mitochondria (the "batteries" inside your cells) so they produce more ATP, the fuel needed for repair and renewal. This extra boost speeds up collagen production, which helps skin look firmer and more vibrant. What's even more exciting is how red light preps your skin to absorb peptides better. When your cells are more energized, they're more receptive to those small, signaling molecules. That means your GHK-Cu or other peptide serums don't just sit on the surface; they penetrate deeper, where they can actually spark change.

If you want to stack your routines for the best payoff, timing matters. Start your morning with a gentle cleanse, then do a red light session for 5–10 minutes while your skin is clean and bare. As soon as you finish, apply a peptide serum or moisturizer to soak in while your skin is warm and receptive. Follow up with your antioxidants (like vitamin C), then layer on sunscreen before makeup. In the evening, after removing the day's buildup, you can use microcurrent or facial massage to stimulate blood flow. Finish with peptides again, locking everything in with a rich cream if your skin feels thirsty.

For those who want to get creative, it is possible to make a DIY peptide sheet mask. Mix a few drops of GHK-Cu serum with a splash of aloe or rosewater, soak a compressed sheet mask in the solution, and lay it over your face after red light or microcurrent. Let it sit for 15 minutes, which gives peptides extra time to work their magic while calming redness and irritation. If you're already visiting a clinic for radiofrequency or laser treatments, talk to your provider about layering peptides afterward; these procedures make channels in your skin that help actives absorb even better, speeding up recovery and boosting results.

Women with more reactive or sensitive complexions will want to introduce new routines gradually, trying one new device or product at a time, and waiting several days before adding another layer. Oily or thicker skin can usually handle stacking treatments more quickly but still benefits from slow increases so your skin's barrier stays healthy. For mature or menopausal skin, moisture is everything; seal in peptides with a nourishing balm after tech treatments to avoid dryness.

If you're further along in your biohacking journey and feeling adventurous, experiment with custom serums, mixing a few drops of peptide concentrate with hyaluronic acid or niacinamide for extra brightening power. Just make sure each ingredient is compatible (avoid mixing acids with copper peptides) and always patch test before slathering it on your whole face. Integrating peptides into clinical procedures can be transformative but should always be done under professional supervision; improper use can cause reactions or waste expensive actives.

Key Takeaways...

Track Progress Like a Pro: Start a photo journal. Take honest, unfiltered shots under natural light every week.

Patience is a Must: Peptides work at their own pace. Don't expect instant miracles!

Expect the Unexpected: Things might stall at some point, and that's okay. If you're not seeing results, check your log for missed doses or lifestyle changes.

Tech + Peptides = Magic: Combine your skincare routine with beauty tech like red light therapy and microcurrent for serious results. These tools help your skin absorb peptides more effectively.

Know Your Skin: Be mindful of your skin type when stacking routines. Sensitive skin needs a gradual approach, while thicker skin can handle more. Mature skin loves moisture, so seal it in after treatments!

SEVEN

PEPTIDE BIOHACKS FOR HEALING, RECOVERY, AND LONGEVITY

It always starts with something innocent: one more rep at the gym, a heroic toddler lift, or just walking like you're not made of glass—and then *bam*, your body files a complaint. You hear that unmistakable *pop* in your knee, or feel a sharp twinge in your shoulder after picking up your youngest (seriously, when did they get so heavy?). These are the kinds of setbacks we've come to tolerate as part of the female experience.

And yes, our bodies are resilient, but let's face it: soft tissue injuries (ACL tears, rotator cuff strains, pelvic floor trauma post-pregnancy) don't exactly roll over and heal with a little rest and rehab. Sometimes, despite all the stretching, foam rolling, and carefully timed yoga sessions, those injuries just won't quit. That's where peptides come to the rescue, not as magic beans, but as powerful little tools that get the healing process back on track.

Take *BPC-157*, for example. This peptide is like your body's personal first responder. Derived from a protein found in human gastric juice, it kicks off the healing process by promoting angiogenesis, aka the growth of new blood vessels. These vessels help deliver the good stuff (oxygen and nutrients) directly to the injured area.

And while most painkillers just slap a Band-Aid on your pain, BPC-157 goes deeper. It helps dial down the swelling without blocking the inflammation you actually need to repair tissue. So, less puffiness and stiffness, without slowing down the healing. Plus, it boosts collagen production, which means your body gets a little help from its trusty fibroblast army, those hardworking cells that repair the tiny tears in your tissues.

Then there's TB-500 (thymosin beta-4), the repair-cell recruiter of the peptide world. It's like the office manager of your body, gathering all the repair cells and sending them to the injury site to get to work. Whether you're dealing with muscle tears, joint sprains, or the aftereffects of childbirth (looking at you, pelvic floor), TB-500 is your go-to. It's also particularly helpful if your healing seems to slow down after forty (hello, perimenopause), thanks to the hormonal shifts that often leave your body dragging its feet in recovery.

So, while peptides aren't *miracle workers*, they're certainly the next best thing when you're looking to speed up recovery without relying on endless rest or masking pain.

If you're considering these peptides, dosing and timing are key. For most women's soft tissue injuries, a typical protocol is:

- **BPC-157**: 250 micrograms injected subcutaneously (under the skin) daily, as close to the injury site as possible. For example, inject near the sore knee, using proper hygiene and a fresh needle every time.
- **TB-500**: 2 milligrams, injected subcutaneously in the abdomen or thigh once weekly.

Both peptides can be used together for 2–4 weeks, starting with daily BPC-157 and weekly TB-500. Store them in the refrigerator after mixing, and use an insulin syringe for accuracy.

To maximize results, combine peptides with intentional movement and smart rehabilitation. The first week after an injury or starting peptides should focus on rest and gentle mobility, like ankle circles for feet or shoulder pendulums for rotator cuffs. As pain recedes (often within 5–10 days), begin stretching and low-impact activities such as swimming or stationary biking.

Follow your physical therapist's guidance, and never push through sharp pain; peptides accelerate healing but don't make you immune to reinjury.

Combining peptides with other therapies boosts results. For swelling, alternate ice and gentle heat (not simultaneously) to improve circulation and reduce stiffness. Some women find that injecting peptides before physical therapy lessens post-session soreness. If you use massage or foam rolling, do these after your injection, when tenderness subsides.

Recovery expectations: Most women notice less pain within a week, sometimes even sooner for milder injuries. By week two, range of motion typically increases. For example, bending a postoperative knee further or moving a formerly painful shoulder more freely. Strength gains usually become apparent by weeks three or four: climbing stairs more comfortably or lifting without discomfort. Pelvic floor healing may take longer; some women experience better bladder control or less pelvic heaviness in two weeks, but a full recovery could take four to six weeks or more, especially after pregnancy.

Immune Support

Navigating daily life means we're constantly exposed to stress, germs, and the invisible wear and tear of modern routines. Your immune system is your built-in shield, working around the clock to keep you safe. But sometimes, that shield feels a bit thin, especially during cold and flu season, after a big project at work, or when you're caring for little ones who bring home every bug from daycare.

Peptides like Thymosin Alpha-1 and LL-37 have surfaced as reliable allies for these moments, supporting your body's natural defenses without overwhelming your system or causing harsh side effects. These are practical tools for women who want to stay resilient and feel strong in the face of constant demands.

Thymosin Alpha-1 works by activating T-cells, the white blood cells that spot and destroy troublemakers like viruses and rogue cells. This peptide also calms overzealous inflammation, making it especially helpful if your system tends to overreact (think flare-ups, allergies, or mysterious aches). LL-37 is more of a frontline warrior with antimicrobial properties, punching holes in bacterial membranes and interfering with viruses before they get a foothold. LL-37 also tweaks cytokine signals, which are like text messages between immune cells, so your response is balanced and not too aggressive.

If you're gearing up for winter or anticipating a stressful stretch (holidays, travel, busy work periods), Thymosin Alpha-1 fits well as a preventive mainstay. A typical protocol involves 1mg injected subcutaneously twice a week for four weeks. Many women use this as an annual "immune tune-up" in early fall or before travel, giving their bodies a subtle boost without overstimulation. It's well tolerated, and you can combine it with your usual supplements. At the first sign of infection (scratchy throat, headache creeping in, or that unmistakable "something's coming on" feeling) LL-37 becomes valuable. A provider might recommend a short burst: 100mcg to 500mcg daily for five to seven days, usually injected subcutaneously in the abdomen or thigh. Always check with your healthcare provider about timing and dosing based on your health history.

Your immune system isn't static, and different life stages

demand different strategies. If you're pregnant or postpartum, the body's defenses naturally shift, sometimes swinging low to avoid overreacting to the baby, other times leaving you prone to lingering sniffles or slow recovery from even minor colds. Perimenopause brings its own quirks: hormone swings can destabilize immune balance, leading to more allergies or odd infections that seemed rare before. Women juggling high-stress jobs or caring for aging parents often notice they're the first to get sick when stress peaks. Even after an intense workout or endurance event, some women find themselves under the weather—this is immune suppression kicking in as the body recovers.

Supporting your immune resilience means creating a lifestyle that works like a well-oiled machine. Think of it like a tag team effort: pair those powerful peptide protocols with a Mediterranean-style diet—hello leafy greens, olive oil, fish, beans, and all the veggies your plate can handle.

And let's talk sleep, because if you're not getting at least seven hours, we need to have a serious chat. Blackout curtains, white noise machines, whatever it takes. If you're not getting quality rest, you might as well be leaving the back door open to every virus that comes along.

Stress management is another big player in the immune game. Mindful movement, like yoga or even just ten minutes of deep breathing, can work wonders for keeping cortisol levels from skyrocketing. Less stress, stronger immunity; it's science, people.

Now, about supplements. They're like the sidekick to your peptides. Vitamin D (1,000–2,000 IU a day) keeps your T-cells sharp, so they're ready to battle any invaders. Zinc (10–25mg) is like your immune system's repairman, fixing everything up when it needs a little TLC. And vitamin C (500–1,000mg) is your antioxidant superhero. If you're traveling or heading into germ-infested zones (like airplanes or crowded events), think about adding elderberry syrup or echinacea for a little extra defense.

And definitely don't underestimate hydration. Water isn't just for making you feel like a glowing goddess; it helps flush out toxins and keeps your mucous membranes nice and moist as your body's first line of defense.

If you're postpartum, keep an eye on your immune system. More frequent sniffles or that lingering cough could be a sign your body's asking for some extra TLC. For those navigating the hormonal rollercoaster of menopause or juggling high-stress work lives, tracking how often you get sick (and how long it takes to recover) can help you know when it's time to launch into an immune protocol versus when a few lifestyle tweaks will do the trick.

Peptide Insights

Pause and ponder immune inventory.

Grab your journal or notes app and track the last three times you felt run-down or got sick. Note what was happening in your life (stressful project? kids back at school?), how long symptoms lasted, and what helped most. Jot down any patterns you spot: maybe colds always hit after big deadlines or during holiday chaos.

Use this information to plan your next preventive peptide protocol and prioritize self-care when you know your system will be tested.

Longevity Peptides

Perhaps we've all wondered, at one point or another, why our skin doesn't bounce back like it used to or why energy doesn't quite spring like it once did. Trust me, a lot of women are on the same page. When all is said and done, it's not about avoiding age, but about embracing it, just with a little extra glow. Who wouldn't want not just more years, but better ones?

That's where longevity peptides like Epitalon and FOXO4-DRI come in, offering a fresh take on aging. They focus on the real business of getting older, not just what you can see in the mirror but what's happening under the hood. These peptides are like VIP bodyguards for your biology, keeping you sharp and resilient by targeting core processes rather than just masking the obvious signs.

Let's talk Epitalon for a second. It's all about those telomeres, the protective little caps on your DNA, kind of like the plastic tips on your shoelaces. They keep things from unraveling, literally. Every time a cell divides, those telomeres shorten, and when they get too short, it's like the biological equivalent of running out of gas. Cells stop dividing, and bam—aging accelerates. But Epitalon? It's like a tune-up for your telomeres. It boosts telomerase, an enzyme that helps rebuild those caps, giving your cells the ability to keep doing their thing for a lot longer.

Using these peptides is relatively simple but should be done with much care. For Epitalon, a typical regimen is 10mg daily for 10 days, repeated twice annually (this is based on Russian clinical protocols). These injections are subcutaneous (abdomen or thigh), done at the same time each day for consistency.

Again, peptides work best when added to a solid foundation of healthy habits. They can't compensate for chronic stress, poor diet, or lack of movement. To get the most benefit, pair peptides with consistent strength training, a nutrient-dense diet (lots of vegetables, healthy fats, quality proteins), restorative sleep (7–9 hours per night), and stress management practices you enjoy (from laughter with friends to peaceful walks). With these fundamentals in place, peptides can enhance sleep quality, mental clarity, skin elasticity, hormone balance, and immune function.

For tracking, commercial biological age tests, such as DNA methylation or telomere analysis kits, can reveal if your cells are aging slower or faster than your chronological age. You can test before starting an Epitalon cycle and again six months later for measurable changes. Simple physical benchmarks like grip strength, walking speed over 20 feet, or standing up from the floor unaided also reflect real-world resilience and improvement.

Women often notice early improvements (better sleep, waking up clearer-headed, smoother menstrual cycles, or reduced brain fog) sometimes after just one Epitalon cycle. Over time, some experience fewer infections and faster recoveries. These are signs of the body working more efficiently when waste is cleared from cells and DNA protection is reinforced.

If you enjoy tracking numbers, DNA methylation clocks (like

Horvath) or telomere length tests are now accessible online. These home kits use a cheek swab or finger prick, letting you track your "cellular age" and see if your healthy routines and peptides are making a tangible difference.

Epitalon has more research and is considered safe at recommended doses, while FOXO4-DRI is still experimental, especially in women. Its potential (clearing senescent cells tied to joint pain, cognitive decline, and more) is exciting, but not yet fully proven. If you're daring and have medical supervision, exploring FOXO4-DRI is possible; otherwise, sticking with well-studied options like Epitalon is prudent.

Monitoring Side Effects

Starting any new protocol that affects healing, immune strength, or longevity can be nerve-wracking. You may wonder what's normal, what's a concern, and how to handle unexpected symptoms. The goal here is to help you feel confident about monitoring yourself, knowing when to pause, and what actions to take if issues arise.

With healing peptides, immune modulators, and longevity stacks, most mild side effects appear in the initial days or weeks. The most typical are mild soreness or redness at the injection site (similar to a tiny bruise), light headache, or temporary fatigue, all of which generally resolve quickly. Some women notice slight swelling or redness near the injection, which usually disappears within hours. Brief cold-like symptoms can occur with immune peptides like Thymosin Alpha-1 or LL-37, and longevity protocols may temporarily affect sleep or mood. These usually aren't cause for concern if they fade quickly and don't worsen.

However, some side effects require immediate attention. If you develop a spreading rash, persistent swelling lasting longer than a day, fever, chills, or chest/throat tightness, stop your protocol right away. Allergic reactions may start as itching or hives, but they can escalate quickly. Other reasons to seek medical help include sudden or severe headaches, ongoing nausea/vomiting, yellow skin or eyes (possible liver issues), unusual bruising or bleeding, pus at the injection site, or a fever over 100.4°F (38°C). Promptly contact your healthcare provider for any of these issues.

Tracking your body's responses is also essential. Keep a daily log during the first week of any new peptide. Each evening, note temperature, mood, fatigue (rated 1–10), any soreness or swelling, headaches, sleep changes, and energy levels. At the end of the week, look for patterns: are things improving, staying the same, or getting worse?

If you experience mild side effects like soreness or headache, pause for one dose and observe. Using ice on the injection site can help, and a pain reliever may be used (avoid NSAIDs unless your provider says otherwise). For temporary fatigue, focus on hydration and rest; often, lowering the dose helps. If symptoms disappear after skipping a dose, resume at half dose for two days before returning to the full protocol. For ongoing mild issues, try reducing frequency (every other day for a week, then every third day) completely stopping if side effects persist.

Some symptoms mean you must stop for good: documented allergic reaction (hives, facial/lip/tongue swelling), fever, severe gastrointestinal issues (unstoppable diarrhea or vomiting), jaundice, chest pain, fainting, or infection at the injection site lasting over 24 hours. Never resume without medical guidance.

If you need urgent medical care, bring your documentation and be direct: "I'm using a peptide called [name] for recovery/immune support/anti-aging. In the last [X] days I've had [describe symptoms], which haven't resolved after stopping the peptide. Here's my log." This helps providers help you more quickly.

. . .

Progress comes from both moving forward and knowing when to pause. Most women experience only minor, brief side effects that fade, but taking prompt action when things feel off protects both your well-being and results. Listening to your body and tracking side effects will keep progress safe and sustainable.

EIGHT
MASTERING THE PEPTIDE LIFESTYLE

Sipping tea, hair in a messy bun, you find yourself phone in hand, scrolling through your health app. I get it. There's a very special kind of satisfaction in watching our sleep scores rise, mood dots shine a little brighter, and those energy crashes spread out like a well-organized calendar.

If you've ever tracked your steps or snapped a progress selfie, you already know that rush of turning invisible changes into visible victories. And with peptides? Oh, it's next level. You're not just hoping for results anymore; you're collecting evidence, learning what your body loves (and what it hates), and figuring out exactly what's working, or what needs a little tweak. Such is the world of biohacking, where *you* are the experiment.

Maximizing peptides is like being your own personal scientist (no lab coat required), just a bit of honest tracking and some serious self-awareness. Start with simple daily logs, as detailed in previous chapters. Record the essentials: energy (1–10), sleep quality (how many hours + how you feel), mood (happy, flat, anxious, sad), and any side effects (headache, bloating, or that random swelling we all try to ignore). If it's relevant, add a note about your menstrual cycle, because that mysterious rollercoaster can explain those weird spikes and dips in your data.

If you're keeping tabs on body composition or skin health, track things like weight, waist/hip measurements, skin hydration (there are affordable gadgets for that), or even hair density. And let's not forget the weekly photo (same lighting, same pose) to catch those subtle changes the mirror just doesn't want to admit.

Choose the tracking method you'll reliably use. Paper works if you love it, but many women prefer digital tools for ease. SHOTLOG is a standout app for peptide users. You can customize cycles, log doses, track side effects, and schedule reminders for injections, hydration, meals, or weigh-ins (Search for SHOTLOG - Peptide Tracker on the App Store). If you already use Heads Up Health, Cronometer, or MyFitnessPal, just layer your peptide notes in. Wearable tech like Oura rings, WHOOP bands, or Apple Health can sync with these apps, letting you see how sleep cycles or HRV change alongside peptide protocols. Suddenly, you'll spot connections, like your best sleep peaking after week three on CJC-1295 or glowing skin following GHK-Cu use.

Some numbers matter beyond feelings or appearances. **Biomarkers** are every serious biohacker's secret weapon. If you're routinely using peptides, track :

- Fasting insulin (aim for <4)
- IGF-1 levels (reflecting growth hormone activity)
- C-reactive protein (CRP) for inflammation
- Menstrual cycle timing (if relevant)

For skin or hair goals, track:

- Hydration (with smart scales or analyzers)

- Hair density (count new hairs in a set patch every few weeks)

You can run these labs before starting a new peptide, then repeat every 8–12 weeks to spot trends early. Start by plotting daily logs against weekly outcomes. If energy dips after raising your dose, adjust or try different timing.

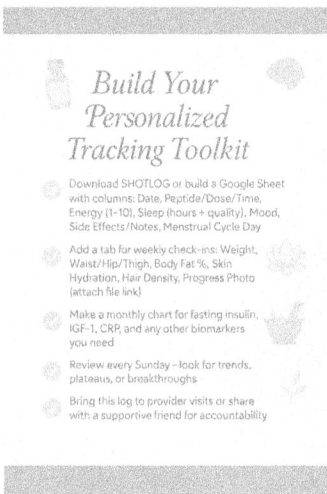

Build Your Personalized Tracking Toolkit

Download SHOTLOG or build a Google Sheet with columns: Date, Peptide/Dose/Time, Energy (1-10), Sleep (hours + quality), Mood, Side Effects/Notes, Menstrual Cycle Day

Add a tab for weekly check-ins: Weight, Waist/Hip/Thigh, Body Fat %, Skin Hydration, Hair Density, Progress Photo (attach file link)

Make a monthly chart for fasting insulin, IGF-1, CRP, and any other biomarkers you need

Review every Sunday – look for trends, plateaus, or breakthroughs

Bring this log to provider visits or share with a supportive friend for accountability

Spot a correlation between better sleep and peptide consistency? Keep it up and celebrate small wins. If CRP or insulin drop after two months, you're making visible health strides. You can even use simple line graphs in Google Sheets or easy mood boards in Canva to visualize patterns and outliers. Bring these charts to medical check-ins; objective data will be appreciated, alongside your experiences.

Recognizing Non-Response

Sometimes, women pour their heart into a new protocol, follow every step, and still feel like nothing's shifting. It's frustrating, especially when they're expecting energy to climb, skin to glow, or even just experience a little less joint pain.

So, how will you know if you're a non-responder to a peptide or just not giving it enough time?

The first hint usually comes from your own experience. After four weeks, check in with yourself: do you feel any difference in the way you move, sleep, or recover? Is your mood steadier? Joints less cranky? If not, don't panic yet; some changes are subtle or build slowly. At the eight-week mark, look for more tangible shifts: maybe improved muscle tone, a lighter step, or even a comment from someone who hasn't seen you in a while. By twelve weeks, if you're still not seeing or feeling any improvement (and your biomarker tests are flat) it's time to call it. This doesn't mean peptides "don't work" for everyone; it means your body might need a different approach.

Non-response can happen for all sorts of reasons, and it's rarely a personal flaw. Sometimes, genetics play the biggest role. Perhaps your body just doesn't have the right receptors in high enough numbers for a specific peptide to work its magic. Absorption can be tricky too; maybe the peptide isn't getting where it needs to go because of poor injection technique or hidden digestive quirks.

Lifestyle also matters more than people assume. High stress, erratic sleep, alcohol, and nutrient gaps can make your system less responsive, almost like trying to water a plant in rocky soil. Even something as basic as low vitamin D, iron, or B12 can blunt results, as these nutrients help peptides do their job. Sometimes, the protocol itself isn't quite right. Maybe the dose is too low for your physiology, the timing is off, or the delivery method isn't ideal for your metabolism.

Troubleshooting non-response means getting curious and systematic instead of frustrated. Start by revisiting your logs to look for patterns or gaps. Did you miss doses? Were there weeks when stress or illness threw everything off? Next, double-check your injection skills. Are you rotating sites? Using clean technique? Hitting the right tissue depth? If you suspect absorption is an issue, consider switching up the delivery method. For example, if injections aren't doing much with GHK-Cu, try a high-quality nasal spray or topical formulation, as different tissues absorb differently for each woman. Protocol mismatch is another culprit; sometimes, stacking peptides can jumpstart a stubborn system.

If all the basics are dialed in and still nothing shifts, adjust your dose within recommended safety limits. For many peptides, this means slowly increasing frequency or amount, or adjusting timing to suit your routine and circadian rhythms. But don't just chase higher doses; sometimes less is more, especially if your body needs a rest or reset.

Of course, if you have underlying nutrient deficiencies, focus on correcting those first, and get bloodwork done if you haven't already. Iron, vitamin D, magnesium, and B-complex vitamins often make the difference between "meh" and "wow." And, if you're still getting nowhere after all this effort, it may be time to switch compounds altogether.

As personalization is your secret weapon here, use responder/non-responder checklists and decision trees to narrow down what's working (or not working) for you. For example, if you've been using GHK-Cu for three months with zero improvement in skin hydration or tone (and your hydration tracker agrees), walk through an audit:

- Are you applying consistently?
- Is the product reputable and not expired?
- Have you tried a different application method?
- Did you pair it with red light therapy or another synergistic biohack?
- Have you checked for deficiencies that could block collagen production?

If every box is ticked and there's still no difference, mark yourself as a likely non-responder for that peptide and move on with zero guilt.

. . .

So, just keep in mind that even science-backed protocols can hit roadblocks due to individual biology. At times, what works wonders for one woman may do little for another. Stay curious and compassionate with yourself as you adapt and experiment. The more precisely you listen to your own data and responses, the closer you get to protocols that fit your life and goals.

When to Cycle Off

Ever notice your workout stops delivering results after a few months? That's your body adapting, and peptides work similarly. This phenomenon, called receptor downregulation, is your body's way of tuning out overstimulation, like an app that freezes when you keep pressing a button too often. Cycling off peptides is comparable to rebooting your device or switching up routines; it refreshes your receptors, prevents plateaus, and keeps results coming instead of causing burnout.

When to cycle off depends on the peptide's purpose.

Fat loss peptides, such as CJC-1295 and Ipamorelin, are typically used for about eight weeks followed by a four-week break, allowing your body to regain sensitivity and reduce the risk of overuse.

Healing peptides like BPC-157 or TB-500 often run for four to six weeks, then pause for two to four weeks if more healing is needed.

. . .

Cognitive and mood peptides such as Selank or Semax are best cycled two weeks on, at least one week off, especially if you notice waning effects.

Longevity peptides (Epitalon, FOXO4-DRI) require less frequent use, usually once or twice a year with lots of downtime.

Immune peptides like Thymosin Alpha-1 should be used carefully and typically under medical guidance, especially if you have significant health concerns. Don't aim for constant stimulation; your system benefits from breaks.

During a "washout" or break, it's common to feel dips in energy, mood, or motivation. These shifts aren't worrisome; it's your body adjusting and recalibrating its natural rhythms without extra signals. You might sleep more deeply, notice increased hunger, or feel tired in the first week off as hormones stabilize. Consider this a biological refresh. Pay attention to your needs: rest, nutritious food, and maybe a few guilt-free naps.

Supporting yourself during these off-cycles by sticking to **healthy basics**. Stay hydrated, aiming for at least half your body weight in ounces of water daily. Prioritize quality sleep with good habits like a cool, dark, screen-free bedroom. Adaptogens, such as ashwagandha or Rhodiola, can help smooth mood swings and low energy without overstimulation. Stick to comforting routines: gentle movement, stretching, walks outside, or slow-paced yoga help both mind and body reset. If structure motivates you, plan and schedule these supportive habits just as you would your peptide cycles.

To maintain benefits during off-cycles, shift your focus to strategies that support your progress without overstressing your system. You can try different supplements, like collagen peptides or omega-3s for joint and skin health, or try lifestyle biohacks tailored to your needs. Off-cycles can be a good time to try red light therapy for skin or breathwork for stress reduction. For ongoing fat loss or muscle gain, try new strength exercises or interval training to keep your body challenged. For cognitive maintenance, try a nootropic tea or a mindfulness practice while you pause Selank or Semax.

Bodies thrive in cycles of work and rest, and the pauses are key to sustained long-term gains. Honor the discipline it takes to pause and reflect on your progress, using this down time to assess what feels truly sustainable going forward.

Your Peptide Network

Exploring peptides can feel lonely, researching protocols and quietly logging progress, often without anyone nearby who truly understands. Yet, real progress rarely happens alone. There's powerful momentum in connecting with others, even virtually.

Look for spaces where women share notes, celebrate wins, discuss research, and solve problems together. Forums like r/Biohackers on Reddit and communities like Biohacker Babes foster open discussion where women talk honestly about cycles, skin, aging, and energy. For expert and peer perspectives, Ben Greenfield's Inner Circle offers science-focused conversations. When joining a group, look for active moderation, clear rules, a mix of scientific talk and personal stories, and a strong stance against hype.

Quality communities cite sources, warn about risky advice, and encourage critical thinking.

Community turns scattered information into collective wisdom. If large forums feel impersonal, start smaller: maybe a private text group or monthly call with a few women you trust. This could include a friend curious about peptides, a sister healing an injury, or a colleague seeking more energy. Your protocols or goals might differ, but what matters is regular check-ins and mutual support. Review results together each month. Sometimes you'll laugh at odd side effects, sometimes brainstorm new strategies, or simply vent about slow progress. This buddy system provides real accountability and motivation when you need it.

Support also means **involving your healthcare team**, even if they didn't recommend peptides. You don't need to master all the science, but do keep them updated. Clear, organized updates show that you're proactive and respectful of their expertise. If you're tracking data digitally, bring summary printouts or screenshots to appointments. Most will appreciate concise, well-organized information that keeps them in the loop.

Sometimes sharing is challenging. You might feel nervous talking about injections with a partner, or worry about skepticism from family who equate peptides with bodybuilding. When discussing with loved ones, stay simple and grounded: "I'm trying something new to help with energy and healing called peptide therapy. I've researched it and am tracking my progress for safety." If pressed with doubts or questions, it's fine to set boundaries: "I'm happy to share what I know, but this is something I'm exploring. If I need your help or advice, I'll let you know." In professional or less personal settings, you're not obligated to give details. A neutral, "I'm working on new wellness habits," is usually enough.

If you're concerned about stigma or being misunderstood, especially around self-injecting or biohacking in general, decide ahead of time what you're comfortable sharing. You could say to a friend:

"I know it sounds unusual, but I've checked out the science. Want to hear why I chose this?" Or, to a skeptical family member: "It's okay if you don't get it; what matters is that I feel better." Some women even prepare a brief info sheet with trustworthy sources for difficult conversations, as sharing facts can often smooth things over faster than debate.

If you ever do feel isolated, please **remember that you're not alone**. Countless women are experimenting, searching for better energy, balance, and health. Connect in online forums, start a local group, or simply lean on one friend who understands. It's easier and more enjoyable when the path is shared.

Peptide Insights

Jot down three people or communities you could include in your support network. Who could you contact during tough weeks or celebrate successes with? What kind of accountability (weekly messages, monthly calls, group progress tracking) feels most motivating?

Finally, set an intention to reach out this month.

_____

_____

_____

_____

_____

_____

_____

_____

_____

_____

_____

Integrating Peptides with Other Biohacks

Finding your rhythm with peptides is less about strict rules and more about blending them into your wellness habits. There's nothing quite like the moment when a woman realizes peptides aren't some all-or-nothing commitment. They're more like a friend who shows up to a party and makes everything better without stealing the spotlight.

So, let's talk about the magic of health combos.

Take CJC-1295 and intermittent fasting, for example. These two combined help your body tap into fat-burning mode while keeping your energy stable. It's like getting the benefits of natural growth hormone pulses from fasting, plus a little peptide nudge to make sure those benefits actually show up. Some women swear this pairing helps them break through stubborn plateaus where diet just can't seem to catch a break.

And then there's BPC-157 for recovery. Want to take it to the next level? Add collagen peptides to your morning smoothie. BPC-157 gets your tissues to repair, and collagen provides the raw materials.

But let's not forget the all-important foundation: sleep. You can have all the peptides in the world, but if you're not getting good rest, it's like trying to bake a cake without turning the oven on. Peptide protocols for recovery (especially CJC-1295 or Epitalon) work their magic best when you're getting proper sleep. So, no need to flip your life upside down; just start small. Create a soothing wind-down routine: dim the lights an hour before bed, sip some calming tea, and banish your phone to airplane mode. Keep your bedroom cool, dark, and quiet. If you struggle to fall asleep, try a magnesium supplement, but steer clear of vitamin C or strong antioxidants at night, as they can mess with some peptide actions. And if stress keeps you awake, a few minutes of slow breathing or a guided meditation can switch your nervous system into "rest" mode, helping mood-supporting peptides like Selank do their thing.

Exercise also fits perfectly into the peptide picture, but timing is key. If you're working on a fat-loss stack, schedule workouts in the morning or early afternoon. Strength training a few times a week works wonders with growth hormone peptides; think muscle gain, fat loss, and faster recovery. For healing protocols, listen to your body. Gentle yoga, a walk, or some resistance bands might be all you need. Don't push through pain or fatigue, that'll just slow down the healing process. For stress reduction, mix in low-intensity movements with breathwork or mindfulness, especially if you're using peptides for mood or brain health.

BENEFICIAL BIOHACKS WITH PEPTIDES

BIOHACK	PEPTIDE	BENEFIT
Intermittent Fasting	AOD 9604	Reduces body fat
Strength Training	Ipamorelin + CJC-1295	Builds lean muscle
Supplements + Meditation	Epitalon	Promotes healthy aging
Bedtime Routine	DSIP	Improves sleep quality
Puzzles + Learning	Dihexa	Boosts brain function
Heart-Healthy Diet	PT-141	Enhances libido

* Usage once daily suggested for all combinations

BIOHACKING FOR WOMEN

Staying Up-to-Date

With new studies emerging daily and peptide trends changing rapidly, staying current can feel overwhelming. It's easy to lose track or feel left behind by all the "breakthrough" headlines. You might feel both excitement and hesitation, wondering, "Is this safe for me?"

Cutting through the noise requires a reliable system. Just 20 minutes a week spent scanning top newsletters and resources can help. SelfHacked simplifies complex science with a skeptical approach, while Examine.com provides deeply researched content, always citing sources and remaining free of product pitches. The PeptideSciences blog offers timely updates on protocols, safety, and regulation changes, which helps avoid issues from shifting laws or shipping rules. For on-the-go learning, try podcasts like *FoundMy-Fitness* with Dr. Rhonda Patrick or *The Life Stylist Podcast,* both of which highlight women's health experts and practical stories rather than lectures. By following these, you'll quickly discern real advances from mere hype.

However, headlines aren't enough; it's important to recognize quality research and the frequent hype masked by marketing. If a new peptide gets buzz, pause before acting. Ask:

- *Was the study published in a peer-reviewed journal?*
- *Was the sample size significant—hundreds of subjects or just a handful?*
- *Was the research conducted on humans or merely animals?*
- *Are side effects reported transparently, or does it sound too perfect?*
- *Who funded the study?*

If any answer is "no" or unclear, be cautious. Watch for red flags in product launches or influencer protocols, such as secret formulas, urgency to buy, or testimonials omitting risks. If you notice a supposed "miracle" peptide few can name, celebrity endorsements without evidence, dramatic before-and-after photos lacking medical details, or pressure to buy from only one supplier, pause and investigate before making decisions. Trust is built over time, so don't let hype rush you.

. . .

Learning is ongoing. The more curious and proactive you are in fact-checking, updating your resources, and sharing, the more confident and safe you'll feel in experimenting. Set a reminder for your weekly science review. Add a podcast to your walk or commute. Stay healthy and informed with your mind open and your standards high.

CONCLUSION

As we reach the end of the first step in your peptide biohacking journey, I truly hope you're feeling the same spark of possibility that so many women have experienced along the way. It's that moment when you realize, 'Wait, I can actually take control of my health?' Because the truth is, you absolutely can. You now hold the keys to your well-being, ready to steer toward a life filled with confidence, energy, and a newfound sense of autonomy. It's your time to take charge, and the road ahead is yours to own.

Take a second and think back to where you started. Maybe you were scrolling late at night, completely drained, wondering if peptides were the miracle you'd heard about, or just another "quick fix" you'd regret. This book was never intended to load you up with jargon and promises that sound like they're from a bad infomercial. My goal was simple: hand you the flashlight, so you could actually see the path ahead and move forward with real, actionable knowledge.

So, if you're walking away from this feeling a little less clueless, a little less isolated, and a lot more capable of making choices for your health, mission accomplished.

. . .

Here's a quick recap of everything you've learned (yes, give yourself a pat on the back, you've earned it):

• You now know exactly what peptides are and how they work in women's bodies.

• You've learned how to find safe, trustworthy sources for your peptides. No more shady mystery vials, and you're not just crossing your fingers and hoping for the best.

• You've figured out how to craft a personalized protocol that fits your life. No more trying to squeeze yourself into someone else's version of "perfect."

• You've got the lowdown on how to track your progress with data, not just wishful thinking. #NoMoreGuessing

• You've explored everything from boosting your energy to burning fat to glowing like a skincare ad, plus all the other incredible benefits peptides bring.

• You've learned how to troubleshoot and adapt.

• You've discovered how to mix peptides with the other habits that matter. (Hint: We're talking about food, sleep, movement, self-care...all the things that make life worth living.)

• And most importantly, you've found the power of community. You're not doing this alone. Not now, not ever.

Now, let's simplify it even more. Here are the cliff notes you can take with you:

• **Vet your peptide sources.** No mystery vials, no shady suppliers. Demand transparency and COAs like it's your second job. Protect your health, your wallet, and your peace of mind.

• **Start slow.** Your protocol doesn't need to be a cocktail of ten different peptides to be effective. Trust me, slow and steady wins this race.

• **Track your progress.** Data is your friend. Use whatever works for you—journals, apps, sticky notes on your fridge.

• **Troubleshoot with patience.** Plateaus and side effects? Totally normal. Take a step back, adjust, and try again. Your body's talking; make sure you're listening.

• **Work with your healthcare team.** Keep them in the loop, bring the research, and treat them like partners.

• **Adapt for your unique life.** Your cycle, your stress, your goals: these are the things that shape how you biohack. Don't try to fit your journey into someone else's mold.

• **Stay curious.** Science moves fast, and guess what? You're allowed to evolve right along with it. Keep learning.

Biohacking with peptides isn't magic pills or miracle cures. Take your time, track your progress, and adjust as your body and goals evolve. If you hit a plateau, if you get stuck, or if you just don't know what's next, go back to your notes. Reach out to your community. Ask for professional help. And, above all, be kind to yourself.

Your story is right there, waiting to be written. I know it can feel overwhelming. Maybe you're still holding onto some doubts about safety, legality, or just whether you're doing it *right*. That's normal.

But here's the thing: You now have the tools, the research, and the lived experience to cut through all the noise and fear. You have facts where there were once only questions. And you've learned that success isn't about perfection, but about starting, adjusting, and asking for help when you need it.

So, what's next?

Maybe it's starting your first peptide protocol. Maybe it's having that honest chat with your doctor. Maybe it's tracking your sleep for a week. Whatever it is, take that first step.

Just before I go, I want to say thank you. Thank you for trusting me with your time, your hopes, and your health journey. My mission is simple: to help women like you feel strong, informed, and truly alive. This process is deeply personal, and I don't take it lightly.

My final wish for you? Walk into tomorrow feeling hopeful and equipped. See aging as an exciting adventure, not something to dread. Know that science, self-care, and the support of other women can open doors you never even knew existed.

Your best days aren't behind you; they're waiting for you, just ahead.

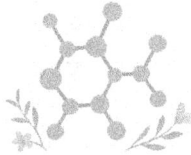

BONUS: TOP 10 MUST-TRY PEPTIDE HACKS

Alright, ladies, if you're ready to hop on the peptide train, here's a list of my all-time favorites that won't leave you scrambling for rare ingredients or drowning in science speak.

These **non-injectable peptides** are your new everyday sidekicks, tackling everything from fighting aging and boosting muscle recovery to giving you that radiant glow.

They're **easy to find**, **simple to use**, and the **results**? Well, they'll speak for themselves.

1. The Collagen Co. – Premium Collagen Peptides

- **Description**: A high-quality, drinkable collagen peptide supplement designed to promote skin elasticity, joint health, and overall vitality. It's perfect for enhancing your body's natural collagen production, which decreases as we age.

- **Type of Peptide**: Collagen peptides (Type I and III)
- **How it is Consumed**: It's available as a powder that can be mixed into water, smoothies, or coffee.

2. Ancient Nutrition – Multi Collagen Protein

- **Description**: This supplement blends five types of collagen peptides into one product, including types I, II, III, V, and X. It's designed to support joint health, skin elasticity, and overall anti-aging benefits.
- **Type of Peptide**: Multi-collagen peptides (Types I, II, III, V, and X)
- **How it is Consumed**: Available in powder form, can be mixed into water, smoothies, or other drinks.

3. Bulletproof – Collagen Protein

- **Description**: Bulletproof's collagen protein is a high-quality, grass-fed collagen peptide supplement that supports skin elasticity and helps with muscle recovery. It also supports gut health, making it a great option for biohacking.
- **Type of Peptide**: Collagen peptides (Type I and III)
- **How it is Consumed**: Powder form, can be added to hot or cold beverages, or blended into smoothies.

4. Organifi – Green Juice with Collagen

- **Description**: A blend of organic greens with added collagen peptides, designed to provide an antioxidant-rich boost while supporting skin and joint health. It's ideal for women looking to improve energy levels and fight signs of aging.

- **Type of Peptide**: Collagen peptides (Type I and III)
- **How it is Consumed**: Powder form, mix with water for a refreshing green juice.

5. Marine Collagen by Further Food

- **Description**: This marine collagen is derived from fish and is perfect for women who want to improve their skin's elasticity and hydration. It's an excellent alternative for those who prefer marine-based collagen over bovine.
- **Type of Peptide**: Marine collagen peptides (Type I)
- **How it is Consumed**: Comes in a powder form and can be mixed into water or smoothies.

6. Cacay Oil – Collagen-Boosting Oil

- **Description**: Cacay oil is rich in vitamins A, E, and F and is known for its skin-rejuvenating properties. While not a traditional collagen peptide supplement, it helps stimulate collagen production naturally.
- **Type of Peptide**: Not a peptide, but acts as a collagen booster for the skin.
- **How it is Consumed**: Topical oil, applied directly to the skin for a hydration boost.

7. The Ordinary Buffet + Copper Peptides 1%

- **Description**: Powerful for supporting skin regeneration by stimulating collagen and elastin production, reduces wrinkles, and promotes skin healing. It's also known for promoting hair growth by reactivating dormant hair follicles.

- **Type of Peptide**: GHK-Cu (Copper Tripeptide-1)
- **How it is Consumed**: Topical application (serums, creams)

8. Swolverine BPC-157 Supplement – The Healing Hero

- **Description**: Known for its regenerative properties, BPC-157 helps accelerate healing for muscle, tendon, and ligament injuries. It also has anti-inflammatory properties and promotes skin and tissue repair.
- **Type of Peptide**: Body Protection Compound (BPC)
- **How it is Consumed**: Oral or topical (creams and serums, but more commonly used in peptide therapy)

9. Life Extension Epithalon – The Longevity Peptide

- **Description**: Epithalon helps promote cellular longevity by activating telomerase, an enzyme responsible for repairing and maintaining the telomeres, the protective caps at the end of chromosomes. This can contribute to a longer, healthier life by reducing cellular aging.
- **Type of Peptide**: Tetrapeptide
- **How it is Consumed**: Oral (capsules or powders)

10. Timeless Matrixyl 3000 Serum – The Wrinkle Reducer

- **Description**: Matrixyl 3000 is a peptide blend that stimulates collagen production to reduce the appearance of fine lines and wrinkles. It enhances skin hydration, elasticity, and tone, making it a powerful tool for anti-aging.

- **Type of Peptide**: Peptide blend (Mainly palmitoyl pentapeptide-4 and palmitoyl tetrapeptide-7)
- **How it is Consumed**: Topical application (serums, creams)

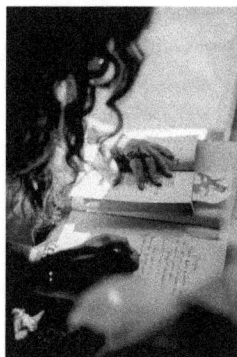

Dear Reader,

Like the other books in this biohacking series, this one was created with women just like you in mind; women who are ready to take charge of their health, not by following the crowd, but by tuning into their bodies and embracing the future of wellness. Women who understand that true vitality comes from a balance of science, nature, and self-trust.

Peptides may sound like something straight out of a futuristic lab, but really, they're the key to unlocking your best self.

So, as you turn this final page, I hope you're walking away with a renewed sense of empowerment. Whether you're balancing hormones, boosting your skin's glow, or optimizing your energy, I truly hope you've seen just how accessible and transformative biohacking with peptides can be.

If this book resonated with you, **I'd be so grateful if you could leave a review on Amazon**. Your voice helps other women on their own journeys of balance and transformation.

Sending you positivity, and a future filled with vitality and grace.

— *Sage O.*

NOW AVAILABLE!

THE COMPLETE
CORTISOL
DETOX
HANDBOOK

A Practical Guide &
Workbook for Balancing
Hormones, Regulating
Emotions, Healing Your Gut,
Reducing Inflammation and
Managing stress

30+
RECIPES
INCLUDED

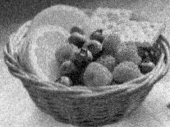

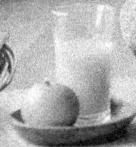

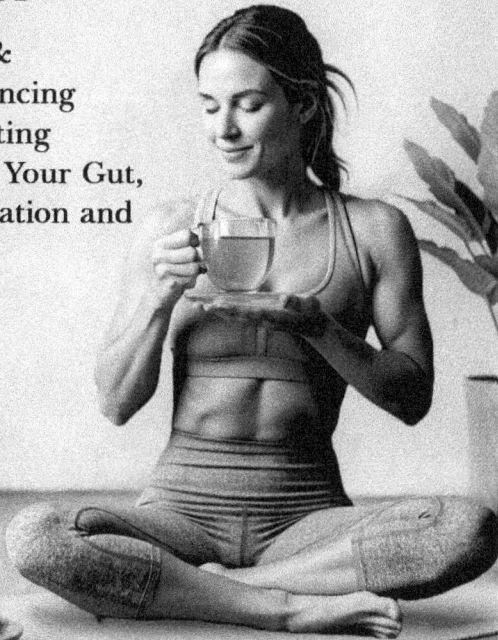

SAGE O'REILLEY

THE EMERALD
S O C I E T Y

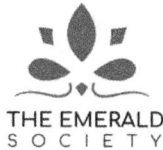

JOIN OUR TRIBE

The Complete Women's Guide to Peptides

Cutting-Edge Biohacking Peptide Therapy to Restore Energy, Balance Hormones, Burn Fat, Enhance Natural Beauty, and Boost Longevity

BIBLIOGRAPHY

- *Peptides: Types, Uses, and Benefits* https://www.webmd.com/a-to-z-guides/what-are-peptides
- *Peptides: Types, Uses, and Benefits* https://www.webmd.com/a-to-z-guides/what-are-peptides
- *Prolonged stimulation of growth hormone (GH) and insulin ...* https://pubmed.ncbi.nlm.nih.gov/16352683/
- *Myths and Facts About Peptide Therapy* https://www.modernwellnessclinic.com/blog/myths-and-facts-about-peptide-therapy
- *Are Peptides Legal? Everything You Need to Know* https://dnlabresearch.com/are-peptides-legal/
- *How to Identify High-Quality Peptides When Shopping ...* https://cdacollaborative.org/pages/how-to-identify-high-quality-peptides-when-shopping-online-in-the-uk.html
- *How to Decipher a Certificate of Analysis (CoA)* https://iris-biotech.de/global/blog/how-to-decipher-a-certificate-of-analysis-coa.html
- *Why You Shouldn't Buy Peptides Online from Research ...* https://revolutionhealth.org/blogs/news/dangers-of-buying-research-pharmacy-peptides
- *Essential Guide to Peptide Dosages: How to Safely ...* https://www.poseidonperformance.com/blog/essential-guide-to-peptide-dosages-how-to-safely-optimize-your-results
- *Essential Guide to Peptide Dosages: How to Safely ...* https://www.poseidonperformance.com/blog/essential-guide-to-peptide-dosages-how-to-safely-optimize-your-results
- *Best Peptides for Women: Fat Loss, Recovery, Skin, and ...* https://swolverine.com/blogs/blog/best-peptides-for-women-fat-loss-recovery-skin-and-anti-aging-benefits?srsltid=AfmBOorbvZ5CPuL2iStaUuXSDomIeu2xK6vKn77MDeteZcAr68-xGqGv
- *Medication Routes of Administration - StatPearls* https://www.ncbi.nlm.nih.gov/books/NBK568677/
- *Peptides for weight loss: Which ones work best?* https://www.medicalnewstoday.com/articles/peptides-for-weight-loss

- *CJC-1295/Ipamorelin Peptide* https://andersonlongevityclinic.com/cjc1295/ipamorelin-peptide
- *GLP-1 Agonists* https://my.clevelandclinic.org/health/treatments/13901-glp-1-agonists
- *Guidelines and Recommendations for Laboratory Analysis ...* https://pubmed.ncbi.nlm.nih.gov/37471273/
- *Peptide Therapy for Women* https://www.bammc.com/women/peptide-therapy-for-women/
- *Functional Connectomic Approach to Studying Selank and ...* https://pubmed.ncbi.nlm.nih.gov/32342318/
- *Intranasal GHK peptide enhances resilience to cognitive ...* https://pubmed.ncbi.nlm.nih.gov/38014118/
- *Peptide Therapy for Menopause - Pure Body Health* https://purebodyhealthaz.com/blog/peptide-therapy-for-menopause/
- *Regenerative and Protective Actions of the GHK-Cu ...* https://pmc.ncbi.nlm.nih.gov/articles/PMC6073405/
- *Is melanotan II safe to use for tanning?* https://www.medicalnewstoday.com/articles/is-melanotan-ii-safe-to-use-for-tanning
- *Multiple potential roles of thymosin β_4 in the growth and ...* https://pmc.ncbi.nlm.nih.gov/articles/PMC7875905/
- *Red Light Therapy and Peptides* https://www.spectraredlight.com/red-light-therapy-and-peptides/
- *BPC 157: Science-Backed Uses, Benefits, Dosage, and ...* https://www.rupahealth.com/post/bpc-157-science-backed-uses-benefits-dosage-and-safety
- *Thymosin alpha 1: A comprehensive review of the literature* https://pmc.ncbi.nlm.nih.gov/articles/PMC7747025/
- *Senolytic Peptide FOXO4-DRI Selectively Removes ...* https://pmc.ncbi.nlm.nih.gov/articles/PMC8116695/
- *Peptides: Types, Applications, Benefits & Safety* https://www.webmd.com/a-to-z-guides/what-are-peptides
- *SHOTLOG - Peptide Tracker on the App Store* https://apps.apple.com/us/app/shotlog-peptide-tracker/id6738789312
- *Biomarkers Every Woman Should Be Tracking* https://www.next-health.com/post/biomarkers-every-woman-should-be-tracking
- *C-Type Natriuretic Peptide Down-Regulates Expression of Its Receptor* https://academic.oup.com/endo/article/146/11/4968/2500301

- *Biohacking for women: What you need to know about ...* https://www.foxla.com/video/1621625

www.ingramcontent.com/pod-product-compliance
Lightning Source LLC
Chambersburg PA
CBHW022057020426
42335CB00012B/729